Praise for Living Well with Bipolar Disorder

"Bipolar disorder can make you feel as if you've lost control of your life. With practical, easy-to-implement wisdom, Dr. Miklowitz shows how to regain a sense of control over this sometimes frustrating, often baffling illness. His insights are invaluable for anyone who has a bipolar diagnosis, or who cares about someone who does. It's rare to find so much clinical expertise combined with such genuine compassion."
> —Terri Cheney, author of *Manic: A Memoir*

"This is an excellent book—a very practical guide to living with bipolar disorder. Dr. Miklowitz, an acclaimed authority in the treatment of mood disorders, provides clear and valuable suggestions for how to navigate a seemingly unnavigable condition."
> —Kay Redfield Jamison, PhD, author of *An Unquiet Mind*

"This is the book I've been longing to read! As a family member of several people with bipolar disorder, I find Dr. Miklowitz's book to be an invaluable resource. He writes with authority, warmth, and compassion. It's the salve every family like mine needs."
> —Meg Kissinger, author of *While You Were Out: An Intimate Family Portrait of Mental Illness in an Era of Silence*

"It is amazing how Dr. Miklowitz takes complex scientific information and boils it down to an accessible guide on how to live with bipolar disorder gracefully. Every conceivable practical aspect of life is covered, from anxiety to sex, from suicidal thoughts to dealing with bosses and coworkers, from combating insomnia to managing anger and irritability. An incredible resource!"
> —Michael J. Gitlin, MD, Department of Psychiatry, UCLA Health

THE GUILFORD LIVING WELL SERIES

The Guilford Living Well Series is designed to help individuals with common psychological conditions solve everyday problems and optimize their quality of life. Readers get specific, empathic advice for stress-proofing daily routines; navigating work, family, and relationship issues; managing symptoms effectively; and finding answers to treatment questions. Written by leading experts on each disorder, books in the series are concise, practical, and empowering.

Living Well with Bipolar Disorder:
Practical Strategies for Improving Your Daily Life
David J. Miklowitz

FORTHCOMING

Living Well with OCD:
Proven Strategies to Take Charge of Your Daily Life
Jonathan S. Abramowitz

Living Well with Social Anxiety
Deborah Dobson

Living Well with Depression
Christopher R. Martell

living well with bipolar disorder

Also from David J. Miklowitz

living well *with*

bipolar disorder

PRACTICAL STRATEGIES
FOR IMPROVING YOUR DAILY LIFE

DAVID J. MIKLOWITZ, PhD

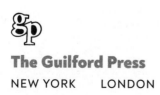

The Guilford Press

NEW YORK   LONDON

Library of Congress Cataloging-in-Publication Data

Names: Miklowitz, David J., 1957– author.
Title: Living well with bipolar disorder : practical strategies for improving your daily life / David J. Miklowitz, PhD.
Description: New York : The Guilford Press, 2024. | Series: The Guilford living well series | Includes bibliographical references and index.
Identifiers: LCCN 2024026576 | ISBN 9781462553532 (paperback ; acid-free paper) | ISBN 9781462555222 (hardcover)
Subjects: LCSH: People with bipolar disorder—Life skills guides. | Bipolar disorder—Treatment—Popular works. | BISAC: PSYCHOLOGY / Psychopathology / Bipolar Disorder | SOCIAL SCIENCE / Social Work
Classification: LCC RC516 .M556 2024 | DDC 616.89/5—dc23/eng/20240724
LC record available at *https://lccn.loc.gov/2024026576*

contents

Purchasers of this book can download and print select materials at *www.guilford.com/miklowitz6-forms* for personal use or use with clients (see copyright page for details).

preface

I have been writing about bipolar disorder since the early 1980s, starting with a set of experiences I had as a psychology intern at the UCLA Mood Disorders Clinic. I was in my early 20s and had lucked into the assignment of running an evening support group for people with bipolar disorder. A good deal of it was focused on how to live a satisfying and productive life despite the disorder. I don't remember much of what I said to the group, but I do remember much of what they said to me. Each person had a distinct story, and each had gone through living hell with bipolar disorder: the hospitalizations, failed medication trials, suicide attempts, and severe family conflicts. They also told gripping stories of exhilaration during mania. Their lives were a lot more terrifying—and a lot more exciting—than mine.

One participant approached me after a group meeting and asked what I did when I went home at night. Did I just go back to my one-room apartment and stare at a single light bulb hanging from the ceiling? When I demurred, he asked, "Who are you exactly, and why are you so interested in us? Are you also bipolar and just hiding it, or does it run in your family or something?" These are questions I've been asked many times since then, usually when people wonder why I am so fascinated by this complex condition.

I have never been diagnosed with bipolar disorder, but there are many things about it that I identify with. The movements of moods up and down, along with subtle changes in sleep and the pace of thought processes. The periods of time when I get irritable or reactive and others when I feel heightened emotion and excitement or dullness and fatigue. Maybe this is just part of the human condition, or perhaps one day we'll learn that it constitutes a subthreshold bipolar condition. In the meantime, though, I continue my fascination.

How This Book Came About

The birth of this book came out of a discussion with my two favorite editors at The Guilford Press: Kathryn "Kitty" Moore and Chris Benton. They had guided my hand through my earlier books, including *The Bipolar Disorder Survival Guide*, now in its third edition. They pointed out to me the need for a book that gives practical solutions for living well with this disorder—not just information but what do you do to prevent episodes and their complications? How do you live your best life despite these dramatic ups and downs? How do you keep symptoms from running your life? In the early part of 2023 we constructed a detailed outline designed to get right to the heart of the matter: answering those questions in the context of daily life within your family and wider community.

My specialization in my research and clinical work is the study of the family —how families communicate, how they solve problems, and, fundamentally, how to help them understand a disorder as challenging as bipolar disorder in one of its members. In every chapter you'll find sections on how to engage your family in helping you deal with this disorder—what is and isn't good for them to do and how to clarify what you need from them. From that vantage point, this book may be as useful for your relatives as I hope it will be for you.

A Word of Thanks

The individuals who have contributed to the content of this book are too numerous to name, but let me highlight several people. My collaboration with Michael Gitlin of UCLA, who was one of my original clinical instructors and continues to be a great colleague and friend, has kept me moving forward in this difficult field. My colleagues in the UCLA Max Gray Child and Adolescent Mood Disorders Program (CHAMP) hold a special place in my heart, including clinical psychologists Patricia Walshaw, Angus Strachan, Sarah Marvin, Marc Weintraub, Megan Ichinose, Danielle Denenny, Alissa Ellis, Lisa O'Donnell, and Jessica Burns; and psychiatrists Elizabeth Horstmann, Robert Suddath, James McCracken, Peter Whybrow, Gregory Barnett, Manal Khan, and Jennifer Nguyen. In addition to being great friends and colleagues, they have helped me train other professionals in how to diagnose and treat young people with mood disorders, and have contributed in immeasurable ways to my research. My staff members at CHAMP, notably the wonderful Georga Morgan-Fleming, Samantha Frey, Brittany Matkevich, Robin Brown, and

Anabel Salimian, have kept the show running and calmed me down when I thought things were going haywire.

My thanks go to Grace Mellor and Seth Patrick Calvin, who contributed art and design ideas for the handouts in this book. Laurie and Steve Gordon have continuously supported my work at the Max Gray CHAMP clinic and have always encouraged me to "think big."

My colleagues in Child and Adolescent Bipolar Network have helped keep the flame alive in an area that seems to be constantly under siege from people who don't believe that kids or teens can get bipolar disorder. These colleagues have, through their writing and research, shown what is and isn't true about bipolar disorder in young people: David Axelson, Melissa Batt, Boris Birmaher, Kiki Chang, Melissa Delbello, Robert Findling, Ellen Frank, Ben Goldstein, Tina Goldstein, Danella Hafeman, David Kupfer, Christopher Schneck, Manpreet Singh, Aimee Sullivan, Eric Youngstrom, and the inestimable Robert Post.

My love and appreciation go to my wife, Mary Yaeger, an artist, who has helped me keep everything in perspective during the long and sometimes arduous process of writing. Your patience and understanding are legendary in our household. My daughter, Ariana, and her husband, Steven Ross, keep me laughing and smiling; and my brother, Paul; his wife, Marija; their daughter, Sabina; and her husband, Alex, have brought joy and reminded me where I came from.

Thanks again to Kitty Moore and Chris Benton, for your insights, rewrites, and good humor. Without you, none of this would have seen the light of day.

Finally, thank you to the numerous people with bipolar disorder and their families I've been privileged to know and treat. Thanks for all you have taught me.

introduction

In the past 20 years, virtually every scientific article I've read about bipolar disorder (BD) starts by saying that the illness is common and impairing, affects 2–4% of the population, and costs the health care system gobs of money. There is usually a statement about its being lifelong and associated with social and work impairments, substance and alcohol abuse, and suicidal thoughts or actions. These articles usually go on to say that we should study some aspect of it (such as genetics, neurological correlates, immunological functioning, or adverse environments) and that doing so will magically lead to the discovery of new and superior treatments. It is rare to see scientific papers address the issue that is most important to people with the disorder and their family members: **What can I do to lead a more fulfilling life despite the illness?**

Despite our best intentions, many people with BD feel let down by the mental health system, whether in the United States or other Western cultures. Mental health care is often cumbersome and inefficient, offering the most services to people who need them the least. People cannot count on getting even the most basic drug treatments for BD from a practitioner who knows what they're doing. And getting psychotherapy for BD, of the type with an evidence base? Too hard to find and, when found, too expensive for the majority of the population.

In the past several decades a number of dramatic first-person accounts of life with BD have appeared, often with expressions of hope. Writers such as Kay Jamison, Patty Duke, Carrie Fisher, Jane Pauley, Terri Cheney, and Gregg Martin lived through incredible challenges posed by the illness, the mental health system, the military, academia, and often their own family members. Most inspiring is how each individual author managed to make peace with the disorder and achieve a balanced life despite seemingly impossible odds. What can we learn from these individuals who have had successful, creative careers and fulfilling family lives despite having severe episodes of mania and depression?

For me, one takeaway from these first-person accounts is that each writer discovered forms of self-care to deal with their illness that went beyond taking medications and attending psychotherapy sessions. They learned to recognize the oncoming signs of new episodes, manage disturbances with sleep, reduce their drive toward drugs and alcohol, and make use of family or friendship supports at times of need. They learned to distinguish who they were as a person from the disorder. It was rarely smooth sailing, but they learned to use their natural creativity, talents, and skills to protect them from the worst of the illness, and learned to lead productive and fulfilling lives. To me, they are the real heroes of our field.

This is a book for people with BD. It aims to fill the gap between the scientific literature and the first-person accounts, to address these questions:

- How can you manage the day-to-day challenges of life with BD?
- How can you have a higher quality of life—with good relationships, satisfying work, and an optimistic view—despite living with this often painful disorder?
- What can you do beyond taking medications?
- What about the problems introduced by medications themselves?
- How can you keep substance abuse from ruling your life?
- How can you maintain good physical health when your moods destroy your motivation to do so?
- How do you explain the disorder to potential partners or employers?
- How can you use family members and friends to help with stability?

If you have BD, you need practical strategies when the inevitable problems of life (some related to the illness, some not) occur. This book is meant to help you at any stage of the illness, whether you're bipolar I or II, a young adult or older, single or partnered, or in your first episode or after multiple episodes have taken their toll.

As you read on, you'll find many illustrations of individuals who have had BD. All of these illustrations are composites—any personal information, including demographic details, has been altered to protect their identities. Nonetheless, their stories exemplify the many ways that people with the disorder have learned to cope and lead fulfilling lives.

How Can This Book Help?

Having BD means you're dealing not only with the stress caused by manic and depressive episodes but also with complicating factors, such as severe irritability, anxiety, suicidal thinking or self-harm, substance or alcohol abuse, and sleep disturbance. You are only too aware of the impact of the disorder on your family members and romantic relationships; your occupational, social, or school goals; and your physical health. You want treatments that are both effective and tolerable, but often struggle to communicate your needs to your doctors or therapists. The solutions you seek require nuanced and strategic thinking.

You may be familiar with another of my books on this subject, *The Bipolar Disorder Survival Guide: What You and Your Family Need to Know, Third Edition* (2019). The two books differ in important respects. The *Survival Guide* explains how the disorder is diagnosed; what is known about it from a genetic, biological, and psychological standpoint; and what medications and forms of psychotherapy are effective in managing depression and mania. The book you're now reading focuses on practical strategies for managing common day-to-day problems. There is much new information in this volume that complements what you already know. If you're newly diagnosed, the *Survival Guide* may be a helpful starting point, but you don't need to have read it to benefit from the strategies recommended in this book.

The solutions offered in this book are sometimes prevention strategies and sometimes things you can do to get through individual moments in daily life without being blindsided by mood symptoms. Sometimes what you can do involves action (such as implementing regular sleep and wake schedules or using certain communication skills) and at other times mindful acceptance (taking a nonjudgmental stance toward problems in the present moment and observing yourself while doing so).

What's the Best Way to Use This Book?

First, start with the "Getting to Know Yourself" section below, which explains a central technique for understanding and coping with BD—tracking your mood states on a mood chart. If you're already charting your moods, you'll have a good idea of what you need right now: help with staving off a looming episode of depression? strategies for when mania threatens to damage your relationships, your finances, or your physical health? tips for communicating with your family members, who mean well but may not know how to help you constructively? With mood charting as the foundation for living well, you can then turn to the chapter that covers the subject with which you feel the need for help—to manage challenges in the present moment or plan ahead for trouble spots that your mood charting history tells you lie ahead.

The book is divided into three parts. Part One, Psychological Challenges: Being Your Own Ally, covers psychiatric symptoms that can really trip you up on a daily basis. It addresses problems that arise during depression and mania, as well as those brought about by the associated features of anxiety, irritability, and suicidal preoccupations. In each chapter you'll find descriptions of typical problems in these areas (often reflected in an anonymous quote from a person with BD), followed by prevention or workaround strategies and how to troubleshoot their implementation.

Part Two, Domains of Life: Daily Routines and Stress, addresses common problems related to physical health, relationships, and career or school objectives. Not being able to sleep can ruin your day, but sleep may elude you because of ongoing mood symptoms and their effects on your circadian rhythms. You may want to get on an exercise routine but find it nearly impossible to do so when depressed. You may want to eat healthily, but your symptoms and your medications make you crave certain foods or drinks. You may have turned to alcohol or drugs to manage or even heighten your mood states (or perhaps you had trouble with substances before you developed BD). Substance abuse and mood disorders are "co-travelers": They can worsen each other, but getting a handle on one of them can also improve the other.

In Part Two, I write about problems that can be caused by family, relationship, and work challenges that both contribute to and are influenced by mood symptoms. Your family may be a source of considerable support or considerable conflict depending on how they respond to your illness and its associated impairments, and in turn, how you respond to your family members. You may be single and interested in finding a new partner, but dating and sex are associated with a different set of challenges, such as how to navigate a new relationship when you're feeling hypersexual, or, in a depressed state, totally uninterested. Even if you're well, when and how do you tell your new partner about your illness? Finally, success in school or the working world can be influenced by the cognitive problems often associated with depression, sleep disturbance, and mood stabilizing medications, but there are things you can do to minimize these difficulties.

Note that many of these problems arise because of people's reactions to you as a person with BD. If your family members think you're inventing your symptoms, they can become frustrated and angry. If your new romantic partner becomes afraid of your mood swings or thinks you're too unstable to sustain a long-term relationship, they may drift away. But there are things you can do, such as educate your family members and partner about your illness, its associated features, and the medications used to treat it. You can use effective communication strategies, acknowledging others' anger or fear while correcting their misattributions about your behavior.

Part Three, Your Treatments: Making the Most of Medications and Therapy, addresses common problems with medication regimens. The majority of people with BD have wondered whether their medications are helping, and many have experimented with going off of them, often with painful consequences. There is no right medication regimen that works for everyone, nor is there only one way to think about it. In this part I emphasize the importance of your agency and choices. You may be with the wrong doctor or taking the wrong medications. You may be able to negotiate a better regimen with your doctor, one that promotes mood stability but also gives you access to your creative instincts. No one should have to tolerate terrible side effects in the name of a balanced mood. In this chapter you'll find a number of strategies for making medication taking more acceptable to you.

Finally, psychotherapy, if available to you, can be a tremendous asset in your overall treatment regimen. It just has to be with the right therapist, one who is open to your goals and uses effective and evidence-based tools. Again, individual choice plays a key role in finding effective psychosocial interventions.

Where Will I Find What I Need in Each Chapter?

Each chapter contains the following elements, although not always in the same order or with the same level of emphasis. I have avoided one-size-fits-all answers. As you'll see, each topic has its own complexities and nuances.

- *Self-assessment.* In each chapter, I encourage you to think about how often or for how long certain symptoms or associated features (such as anxiety and self-harm) occur and whether they vary along with the ups and downs of your mood state, as indicated by your mood charting. I also encourage you to think about the stressors that cause day-to-day variability in these areas. This book shows you how to make the best use of the information you collect.

- *Prevention and in-the-moment strategies.* Sometimes you can take concrete steps to head off a developing problem (such as catching mania in its earliest stages and implementing prevention strategies). At other times you can do something immediately to reduce the impact of current symptoms on your day-to-day life, what we call "harm reduction."

- *Troubleshooting tips.* When the recommended solutions are not working or are too hard to pull off, what kinds of workarounds can you consider? For example, if you find mood charting a drag, there are different ways to do it that don't involve pulling out a written diary every day. If your doctor has recommended exercise but your depression makes it impossible to stick to a structured routine, you'll learn alternate ways to be physically active and stay healthy.

• *Advice on how to engage your family members, partner, or close friends in helping you solve disorder-related problems.* You will find it empowering to have ways to explain your mood swings, anxiety, or job or social problems to your family, specifying the kinds of help that will be of maximal benefit to you. When they say things that you find upsetting or demeaning, there are ways to understand their point of view without giving up yours, as well as ways to explain why things they've said or done are hurtful. Using the skills suggested in each chapter can lead to much more productive and healing interactions with your family or spouse.

• *Fillable charts that will help you organize your use of new skills.* Many of these handouts are time-tested components of family-focused therapy (FFT), the treatment my colleagues and I developed at the University of California, Los Angeles (UCLA). FFT is an effective therapy in combination with mood-stabilizing medications for adults and adolescents with or at high risk for developing BD.

• *Taking stock.* These final sections give you a chance to assess which strategies in the chapter are working for you and which you haven't found helpful so that you can plan for challenges that lie ahead.

A Word about Terminology

There are some terms used frequently in the book that require definitions. First, I use "they/them" pronouns so that no assumptions are made about the gender identity of the hypothetical person I'm discussing. Second, I refer to "your doctor" when I'm talking about the person who is prescribing your medications. Ideally, this is a psychiatrist with training in mood disorders, but in today's medical climate it can also be a general practitioner (GP; sometimes called a *family doctor* or an *internist*) or a nurse practitioner; in some U.S. states it can be a clinical psychologist with prescription privileges. Psychiatrists usually have much more training than other professions in the nuances of prescribing medications, and BD is clearly within their scope of practice. GPs and nurse practitioners can prescribe psychiatric medications, but many feel uncomfortable when the regimens become complex or there are many side effects, and usually will defer to a psychiatrist in such cases.

Third, when I mention "your therapist," this is usually a clinical psychologist, a social worker, a nurse practitioner, or (less common nowadays) a psychiatrist whose main goal is to address the life issues that go along with BD. Sometimes the prescribing provider and the therapist are the same person, although this is infrequent in overburdened community health settings.

I refer to drugs as mood stabilizers (such as lithium, valproate [Depakote], or lamotrigine [Lamictal], the latter two of which are also called *anticonvulsants*), "second-generation" antipsychotics (such as olanzapine [Zyprexa], risperidone [Risperdal], aripiprazole [Abilify], quetiapine [Seroquel], lurasidone [Latuda], lumateperone [Caplyta], or cariprazine [Vraylar]), to be distinguished from the older line of antipsychotics like Thorazine or Haldol; and antidepressants (selective serotonin reuptake inhibitors [SSRIs] like fluoxetine [Prozac] or escitalopram [Lexapro], or serotonin and norepinephrine reuptake inhibitors [SNRIs] like venlafaxine [Effexor]). These classes are named for the condition in which the medicine was first studied, but such names don't necessarily mean anything about the purpose of its use for a given set of psychiatric symptoms. People sometimes assume that if you take an antipsychotic, you must therefore be delusional or have hallucinations. This is not the case, because antipsychotics can be used to treat depression, anxiety, sleep disturbances, and agitation. Antidepressants are not only used for depression; they can be used for anxiety conditions or pain. Anticonvulsants like lamotrigine have mood-stabilizing properties, even though their initial purpose was to control seizures in epilepsy. I give more detail about these medicines in the later chapters.

Navigating Your Own Path

BD is painful and unpredictable, but using the strategies in this book puts the reins in your hands so that you can function at an optimal level in your day-to-day life. I encourage you to get whatever help you need from your doctors (by being informed and assertive when necessary) and your support system (your family, partner, friends), without giving up your independence. My wish is that you will navigate your own unique path in living well with this disorder every day.

Getting to Know Yourself through Mood Charting

One of the most fundamental and important strategies for living well with BD is to keep tabs on your moods and how they interfere with your functioning. The best tool for gathering these insights is the *mood chart*, a diary or calendar for tracking the ups and downs of your mood symptoms. It's more than just tracking whether you feel happy or sad on any given day. The daily ratings incorporate shifts you may feel in your energy levels, thinking, sleep, and behavior—all dimensions relevant to episodes of BD.

Mood charting will be relevant, in various forms, to all of the chapters in this book. If you've been charting your moods for a long time, you may be able to skip the rest of this chapter, but if you've ever had trouble with the consistent use of mood charts, you'll find helpful troubleshooting tips after the instructions for using the charts.

Knowing how your moods and certain problems with daily life interact is key to identifying which strategies in the book will be most helpful. It can do the following:

- Help determine the level of care you need
- Help you identify the early stages of new episodes, which is often the time when you have the most leverage for avoiding a lengthy period of illness or a hospital stay
- Provide your physician with a visual representation of your recent shifts in mood, which can inform changes to your medication regimen
- Reveal whether a new medication has shifted your pattern of mood swings or alleviated a chronically depressed state
- Clarify the role of environmental stressors in triggering mood swings, which can be helpful for your psychotherapy and for preventing future episodes
- Help you evaluate the effects of changes to your daily or nightly routines on your mood states

Basics of Mood Charting

If you're not already charting your moods, start by keeping a weekly chart for the next 2 months, which will give you valuable information as a prevention tool. Once you've found the optimal way to do it, make it a habit and chart as often as you can. The rest of this chapter helps you figure out what actions to take right now if charting shows that your moods are heading into depression and mania. It also suggests strategies for how to make mood charting effective and easy if you're having trouble.

On page 10 you'll see a typical mood chart, which you can complete by simply placing an X on the line corresponding to your mood state (described with the words on the left, or any other words you choose) and the day of the week. You will probably find it easiest to make one mood rating in the morning and another in the evening. If you don't think your moods shift much, you may be able to just make one daily rating, but most people do experience some variation during the day, often feeling worse in the morning and better in the evening. If you have bipolar, mixed periods, with symptoms of mania (*M*) and depression (*D*) co-occurring in the same day or week, make separate *M* and *D* ratings for each day. By the end of each week you should have a graph of the up and down movements of your mood over 1 week. Try to keep the chart for at least 2 months, which will give you a sense of the direction your moods are taking and how much they vary from one day or week to the next. Later you can add other important variables to the chart, such as stressful events or changes to your medications. You can photocopy the blank chart that follows or print copies from the Guilford website (see the box at the end of the table of contents).

Numbers and Words: Tools for Rating Your Mood and Functioning

Following are general descriptions of the points on the left side of the chart—not every example will fit you. Think of these descriptors as temperature readings; not every warm or cool day has the same characteristics. The idea is to characterize not only your moods but also the behaviors that go along with them in the domains of thinking, sleep, energy levels, sex drive, motivation, and other features.

The chart uses a 7-point mood scale that goes from –3 (*very depressed*) to +3 (*severely manic*), with 0 representing your most balanced mood, when you're not feeling high or low. This is what is normal for you. If you are at 0, your sleep is fairly consistent and you've been able to carry out your work or other daily tasks without extra effort. If you're having trouble defining this state, think of how you felt before you developed the disorder, or perhaps how you've felt in between manic and depressive episodes. One fundamental goal of this book is to learn some strategies for keeping your mood up at this balanced level.

DEPRESSION RATINGS

–1 (Mild)

This rating means the following:

- You feel somewhat pessimistic, self-critical, or negative about things.
- You want to sleep more and are having trouble getting out of bed in the morning, but not necessarily every day.

MOOD CHART

Week of _____

Mark your mood for each day with an X, or if you prefer, make one mood rating for the morning and another for the evening.

	Monday	Tuesday	Wednesday	Thursday	Friday	Saturday	Sunday
Severe mania (+3)							
Moderate mania/hypomania (+2)							
Mild hypomania (+1)							
Balanced (0)							
Mild depression (-1)							
Moderate depression (-2)							
Severe depression (-3)							
I woke up at:							
I went to bed at:							
Other observations:							

- Your energy level feels low, even though you can still exercise, walk the dog, or do other physical activities that are typical for you.
- Things may not seem interesting to you; invitations from friends make your mind go to "Do I really want to do that?" You don't enjoy social events as much as usual.
- Your depression may not be obvious to others because your work or school performance has not changed, but if you are married or in a regular relationship, your partner has probably noticed.

≫ Use –1 as your baseline if you always feel mildly depressed, as some people do.

–2 (Moderate)

This rating is reserved for moderate states of depression:

- You feel sad much of the day, hopeless about the future, and slowed down or fatigued.
- You have trouble falling asleep or staying asleep almost every night, or sleep more than your usual (10 or more hours).
- You ruminate about things that happened a long time ago.
- You feel irritated by others, even when they're just trying to be friendly.
- You miss at least a day of work or school each week, or part of a day, and feel much less productive than usual.
- Suicidal thoughts cross your mind.

Others have probably commented that you seem morose, slow, or just withdrawn.

≫ Contact your doctor and therapist, because you may need to adjust your medications, or, at minimum, get more emotional support.

–3 (Severe)

This rating is reserved for severe states of depression:

- You have a numb feeling, in which nothing seems interesting and even basic tasks like taking a shower seem impossible.
- You spend long periods of time sitting in a chair (or lying in bed) and ruminating.
- Your thoughts go slowly and you can't make decisions.

- You have more frequent thoughts of suicide and think about various methods, or you have self-harmed or made an actual attempt.
- You feel like you're being punished.
- You miss multiple days or weeks of work or school.

» You should definitely see your treatment providers if you've had more than 1 day like this.

HYPOMANIA AND MANIA RATINGS

On the flip side are the various stages of hypomania or mania.

+1 (Mild Hypomania)

This mild rating refers to periods of being sped up without impairment in your personal or work functioning. You may be somewhat more productive at work or school. At a +1 rating, you may notice the following:

- You probably feel giddy, cheerful, or, alternatively, irritable and impatient, but it's in the context of everything seeming faster.
- You are more energetic and self-confident, with lots of ideas.
- You have wanted to see and talk to many different people. You may be calling people at various times of the night.
- You may be sleeping somewhat less than usual (as in 5 hours/night) but you don't feel tired during the day.

» You are not in the danger zone, but be aware of the likelihood of escalation.

+2 (Moderate Elevation)

The moderate rating is on the border between hypomania and mania (that is, being wired to the point of being impaired in your functioning):

- You feel very goal driven (wanting to get a lot of things done) or you are much more activated, doing many different things without particular goals in mind.
- Your mind is racing, and you feel much smarter and more insightful than usual.
- Others say your speech is faster and your ideas are coming out too quickly for them to follow.

- You have had run-ins with people (such as coworkers who find you aggressive or overly sarcastic).
- You have had negative exchanges with strangers that are over the top for you (like yelling or cursing at someone who is taking too long to park their car).
- Everyone else seems slow and uninteresting, and you may be irritated when they interrupt your verbal flow.
- You may have an increased sex drive.
- Your sleep has definitely decreased to 4 hours or less, and your sleep may be fitful. You do not feel tired.

» At this point you should definitely have consulted your doctor and, in all likelihood had an adjustment of your medications.

+3 (Severe Mania)

This rating is for severe or "florid" mania. This means the following:

- You are laughing nonstop or extremely giddy and silly, or very angry or enraged.
- You have had severe arguments with others, which may have become physical, or you have wanted to hit people. Others say they can't be around you.
- You are filled with ideas of brilliance, creativity, and talent, or feel like you have special powers or abilities.
- You have become preoccupied with projects that to others seem unfeasible and unrealistic.
- You have done things that are dangerous or impulsive, like driving excessively fast, spending excessively, or gambling money you don't have.
- You have had run-ins with the police or been hospitalized.
- You are not sleeping at all or sleeping very little, and feel no need for it.

» This is a dangerous state, and you and your family need to consider emergency treatment (see the next section).

TROUBLESHOOTING: "I can't figure out which ratings to choose; how do I get this right?"

Because these descriptors include mood, thinking, and behavior, it may take some practice to get used to rating them each day. In choosing your daily or nightly ratings, try to remember how you've felt when you were at your highest of highs or lowest of lows. You may not have experienced the extreme (+3 or –3) ends of the scale. If you have bipolar II disorder, you probably have never gone above a +2 or even a +1 on the mania/hypomania side.

It may also help to compare your mood today with how it is when you're feeling well or balanced. What are you ordinarily able to do that you are finding harder now? How confident do you feel today compared to usual?

Rating Your Sleep

Tracking your wake times and bedtimes will clarify how your sleep and mood are intertwined, which can be different for each person. It's easiest to remember to complete the chart shortly after you wake up. So, for Friday, mark what time you went to bed Thursday and woke up Friday. If you're unsure of what time you woke up, use the time you got out of bed. If you took one or more naps that day, list the number of hours of napping in parentheses next to your wake time.

There are spaces below your bed and wake times for other daily observations, such as:

- If you forgot your medications on one day, record it below the relevant day.
- If you had therapy on a different day, record that.
- If you are keen to record stressors (such as significant arguments with your spouse), record those here in brief.

 TROUBLESHOOTING: "Mood charts don't help me—
I do them for a week or two and quit. What else can I do?"

WORKAROUND 1: Modify the form to make it work for you

There are several things you can try if the methods above aren't working for you. First, consider whether the –3 to +3 scale is too simple or just doesn't capture the movement of your moods, thinking, and behavior from one day to the next. You may feel that a 10-point scale (–5 to +5) fits better, or perhaps you'd rather label the whole dimension as "energy level" or "activity level." If the terms *manic* and *depressed* do not resonate with you, then think of other ways to label the 7- or 10-point scale. Some people describe mania as chaotic, wired, amped, or buzzed. As mentioned earlier, you can depict mixed states by making a mania and depression rating for the same day. Depression may be termed the *blues, misery, gloomy,* or, as many of my patients have said succinctly, "feeling like shit."

WORKAROUND 2: *Try an online mood chart*

If you prefer to fill out a chart online, you can find the chart above at *www.semel. ucla.edu/champ/downloads-clinicians*. Alternatively, you may want to try one of the many commercial apps for rating moods. Examples are Emoods (*https:// emoodtracker.com*), the Depressive and Bipolar Support Alliance Mood Tracker (*www.dbsalliance.org/wellness/wellness-toolbox/wellness-tracker*), or MoodFit (*www.getmoodfit.com*). You can also browse through the list of apps on VeryWell-Mind.com (*www.verywellmind.com/best-mood-tracker-apps-5212922*). These apps have the advantage of tabulating the ratings for you so that you can look at your progress graphically over several weeks. The apps usually send text reminders if you haven't rated one or more days. You still have to make daily mood ratings, but you may find these to be easier than a paper-and-pencil chart.

WORKAROUND 3: *Create your own chart*

Many people start charting their moods and get tired of it, finding it too reduction-istic. You may feel that it doesn't capture the psychological or interpersonal issues that contribute to your mood swings. These reactions are entirely understandable. The best solution is to consider what did and didn't work for you when you tried charting before, why you stopped doing it, and what kind of chart would be more to your liking. You don't need to be a programmer to do this. You can simply keep a diary with descriptions of what stands out about a particular day (such as "fight with partner"), how your mood fluctuated ("angry at first and then depressed"), and how long the mood state lasted ("like 3 days"). Come up with your own way of describing its severity. If you are a visual person, think of a way to graph this information over the next week.

A caveat: Don't try to track everything (your mood, irritability, anxiety, drug or alcohol use, sleep, stress, family arguments, medications, exercise, and eating habits) at once. It's much easier and more useful to track your mood and one or two other daily routines (such as sleep/wake times and medications) and observe their patterning over time. Later, you may want to track your mood in relation to can-nabis use (for example, do you feel down and then get high, or do you get high first and then start to feel more activated?), or your sleep in relation to exercise. Doing so for a month at a time will reveal patterns that you may not know have existed.

Mood charting is the first step in gaining more control over the cycling of your disorder. Now that you know these basics, let's move on to one of the most challenging aspects of BD: dealing with depression.

PART ONE

psychological challenges

BEING YOUR OWN ALLY

Depression and mania, the two central symptom states in BD, go along with various *associated features* (the term used in the *Diagnostic and Statistical Manual of Mental Disorders, Fifth Edition, Text Revision* (DSM-5-TR), all of which can impair your quality of life: severe anxiety and worry, anger and irritability, and suicidal thoughts or impulses. Medications only go so far in gaining control over these features of BD. What can you do yourself, and with the help of your family members or friends, to live the life you want to live? How can you be your own ally?

The premise of this book is that you have more control than it may appear in managing the most difficult parts of your disorder, beyond simply taking medications. In this part, you'll learn how self-management strategies can be brought to bear on the symptoms you experience on a day-to-day basis.

1

depression

PREVENTION AND COPING STRATEGIES

"Mania is the exciting, Hollywood-ized part of this disorder. Unfortunately, depression is what I have most of the time."

—*35-year-old woman with bipolar I disorder*

For most people, depression is the hardest part of BD. For some it comes and goes in episodes of several weeks or months, and for others it is constant. It makes it hard to enjoy even your favorite people or activities. Your medications will help (if they are the right ones), and physical and social activity will lift your mood further. But for many, depression is a "slow burn" that doesn't lift easily. Your mind and body may refuse to cooperate with the demands of the day: You may experience changes in appetite, feelings of guilt or worthlessness (sometimes with thoughts of suicide or self-harm), fatigue, a slowing down of your movements and speech, trouble concentrating, and insomnia. It is hard to explain to others who haven't experienced it. Your parents or spouse are probably confused as to how to help you in this state and, in their confusion, may do or say things that you find irritating.

Is there anything you can do? Yes. In this chapter you'll learn medical and behavioral strategies for dealing with depression in its early phases (to prevent it from getting worse) and how to cope when you're in the midst of it. There are things you can ask of your family members and doctors that will help further. Implementing these strategies will not necessarily prevent depression altogether but they will almost certainly reduce its harmful effects and improve your quality of life. There is good reason to be hopeful.

Prevention Strategies for Depression

When you're feeling OK and have been well for a couple of weeks, there are strategies you can use to prevent new depressive episodes from starting. The same strategies are also helpful if you have had mild depressive symptoms and want to stop them from getting worse. If you aren't sure how best to characterize your current mood state, consult your mood chart (see page 10).

PREVENTION STRATEGY 1: Consider a change in medications

If you're already taking medications for BD, you probably know that they are intended to reduce your current symptoms and prevent future episodes. If you are largely *recovered* from a recent depressive episode—with no or only mild symptoms for the past 2 months—you're in the "maintenance phase" of treatment. The goal of treatment in this phase is to keep you stable and relatively symptom-free, with as few medication side effects as possible. But could more be done to prevent future recurrences? Mood stabilizers like lithium, lamotrigine (Lamictal), and valproate (Depakote), or second-generation antipsychotics (SGAs) like cariprazine (Vraylar) and lurasidone (Latuda) are all used to reduce current symptoms *and* reduce the chances of having new episodes. Dosages of lithium have to be in the *therapeutic range* (usually defined as blood tests with levels of 0.6–1.2 mEq/L [milliequivalents per liter]) to prevent mood episodes.

>> Discuss your current medications and dosages with your doctor.

STRATEGY 1A: Optimize your mood stabilizer

Even if you're stable and have only mild symptoms, you might be feeling sluggish and sedated and still experience mood shifts. In those cases, the best dosage for you could be lower or higher than what you're taking. The therapeutic dosage of lithium varies widely among individuals and needs to be reached gradually. Sometimes lithium causes nausea at therapeutic dosages, in which case an extended-release form of lithium or a once-a-day dosing plan may be better for you.

>> Talk to your doctor about dosages and extended-release plans. Also see Chapter 13 for more on the side effects of mood stabilizers and how to control them.

STRATEGY 1B: Add or substitute a different agent

As you'll read throughout this book, medications that are hard to tolerate or that are not doing their job can be modified through dosage changes or through adding or switching to a different agent. Lamotrigine (Lamictal) is often recommended during maintenance care because it is easier to take than lithium. It appears to be more effective in preventing depressive than manic episodes and is often recommended for people who are "depression predominant," meaning that depressive episodes outnumber manic or hypomanic episodes. Many people with bipolar II disorder fit this qualification. The reverse is true for lithium.

Certain of the SGAs are recommended either as adjuncts to mood stabilizers or as solo agents:

- Lurasidone (Latuda) is increasingly recommended for bipolar depression.
- So is quetiapine (Seroquel), which has clear experimental evidence for prevention of depression.
- The olanzapine (Zyprexa)–fluoxetine (Prozac) combination, also called Symbyax, is prescribed less frequently but has also been shown to prevent bipolar depressive episodes.
- Medications meant to regulate blood sugar (such as Metformin) often are prescribed alongside of SGAs because of the latter's risk of weight gain and sedation.

» Work with your physician to prevent or treat residual symptoms of depression during the maintenance phase.

STRATEGY 1C: Add an antidepressant

If you've been suffering from depressive episodes that have not been alleviated by an optimized dosage of a mood stabilizer or SGA, an adjunctive antidepressant may help you. Antidepressants have some risks: They have been associated with rapid switches from depression into mania or hypomania and "rapid cycling" (the occurrence of four or more mood episodes of any type in a single year). *This risk is mainly among people with BD who take antidepressants without an accompanying mood stabilizer or SGA.*

» Ask your doctor about trying an antidepressant while staying on your current mood stabilizer or SGA. Usually, you would start with a low dose and increase it gradually so that your side effects can be monitored.

The SSRIs are beneficial in preventing and treating bipolar depressions. Other agents, such as bupropion (Wellbutrin) or venlafaxine (Effexor), work in a somewhat different way than SSRIs and may be recommended instead of (or in combination with) SSRIs.

>> Ask your doctor if you should stay on an antidepressant that worked well during your last depressive episode, rather than stopping it. It may help you stay episode-free for longer periods. Make sure your doctor sees your mood chart, and be prepared to describe your pattern of symptoms over the past month. If your mood states have been mainly depressed but there have also been a lot of ups and downs (mood instability), taking an antidepressant is riskier.

PREVENTION STRATEGY 2: Try mindful meditation

Think of depression as your body's and mind's way of telling you that they're exhausted and need a period of rest. One patient of mine described it as "going into your cave and licking your wounds." Rather than chasing it away, try to learn what depression is telling you: What issues in your life are being stirred up? Mindfulness meditation is a way of observing your thoughts and emotions from a distant, non-judgmental, and "decentered" vantage point. This practice can help stabilize your mood when you're depressed and also help prevent future episodes.

STRATEGY 2A: Build a regular meditation practice

Mindfulness meditation practice involves taking 30–60 minutes each day to sit in quiet reflection, focusing your attention on your breathing and experiencing physical sensations like the feeling of your stomach moving up and down. You can do this with your eyes open or closed. Think of the air going in and out of your lungs as being like waves: each building, cresting, and breaking. For now, avoid trying to change the pace or depth of your breathing and instead experience it as a natural bodily function. It's often best to start with 15 minutes a day (many people prefer morning) every few days and gradually build up to 30–60 minutes every day.

STRATEGY 2B: Treat negative thoughts as just passing events in your mind

If you get caught up in the negative thoughts and pessimism that go along with periods of depression, try the following: Sit quietly and allow the negative thoughts to come while being aware of your breathing. You can start to imagine your thoughts as like individual leaves going down a stream, with one not that much different from the other. Be curious about them and ask yourself questions like

"I wonder what made me think of that now?" Take a nonjudgmental, observing stance toward them rather than trying to challenge them or make them go away.

STRATEGY 2C: Don't worry about whether you're doing it right

As you sit, you may feel impatient, with questions like "What am I supposed to be thinking about?" or "I can't imagine my thoughts being like leaves." You're not supposed to be thinking about any one thing—just observe your mind wandering about. If you find yourself getting upset, gently return your attention to your breathing. Meditation is like building muscles—the more regular you are about doing it, the more it will feel like a natural activity.

>> Meditation practices can be a useful strategy in many different situations, and they are recommended throughout this book, so it's worth starting a mindfulness practice now.

>> There are many resources, online and in print, that provide instructions in mindfulness meditation practice, some designed specifically for use with depression, such as *The Mindful Way through Depression, Second Edition* (Mark Williams and colleagues, in press) or *The Mindful Way Workbook: An 8-Week Program to Free Yourself from Depression and Emotional Distress* (John Teasdale and colleagues, 2014). Both books include prerecorded mindfulness exercises that you can listen to on your phone or tablet. There are also a number of self-guided meditation apps that you can download for free (such as the UCLA Mindful app, available at the Apple App Store and Google Play).

PREVENTION STRATEGY 3: Behavioral activation exercises

One of the most powerful things you can do to prevent depression or cope with it when it's present is to stay active, with pleasurable (or at least stimulating) activities. On the surface the premise is simple: Depression goes along with social and physical withdrawal, and when you withdraw you'll experience less reward from your environment, which maintains your depressive state. Reaching out to others and planning your day around activities that give you pleasure will help lift your sadness and anxiety and distract you from the thoughts that go along with them. Of course, this is easier said than done.

When you're well, you can build social stimulation and physical activity into your daily routine, and doing so can go a long way toward boosting your mood (see Chapter 10). Plan a variety of activities for your downtime to help give your day more structure (see the activities list on the facing page), which will make you less vulnerable to a depressive recurrence. But when you're in the midst of a depressive state, you'll need to have a plan for pursuing stimulation and activity at a less demanding level, doing what you can without expecting as much of yourself.

Here are the steps for building an activation plan:

1. When you are feeling well, make a list of activities you could imagine doing when depressed. Try to prioritize activities that involve other people, that occur outdoors, that you enjoy, and, when possible, that involve some degree of physical activity, even if it's just walking to an event. We know that exercise lifts mood even though it can be one of the hardest things to do when you're depressed (Chapter 10).

2. Rate how much mood improvement you predict you will get from each of these activities.

3. Put together a calendar with pleasurable or stimulating activities scheduled for different times of the day.

4. Don't expect to be able to follow through on all of them, but do keep a record of which activities you were able to do and what mood benefits you got, either on your mood chart or in a separate table (see the sample behavioral activation record on the facing page).

 ## TROUBLESHOOTING: "What if I can't get myself to do these things?"

WORKAROUND 1: *Push on through*

Don't wait for the motivation to do these activities. Try to push yourself to do them even though they feel hard, and you may be rewarded with immediate improvement in your mood and energy level. Try to keep this going each day and build on it gradually.

WORKAROUND 2: *Plan the week ahead*

During the weekend, plan out your week with reminders on your phone or on a written calendar. If other people are involved, make arrangements with them in advance, as this will help motivate you to get out.

WORKAROUND 3: *Be realistic about your limits*

Make sure you don't end up doing too much in any one day. It's important to build up to a stimulating day and not neglect rest and sleep.

1. Go to a sporting event.
2. Go to a museum.
3. Play cards with another person.
4. Talk on the phone.
5. Work on a hobby (for example, beading/embroidery, practicing a musical instrument).
6. Do an art project.
7. Go out to eat by yourself or with someone else.
8. Take a bath.
9. Play with a pet or go to a pet shop.
10. Do some "pleasure reading" (that is, unrelated to work or school).
11. Cook/bake something new.
12. Do a puzzle.
13. Go for a drive.
14. Attend a yoga class.
15. Go see a local band performance.
16. Go to a movie.
17. Shoot some pool.
18. Go to a coffee shop.
19. Go on a day hike.
20. Do some gardening.
21. _____
22. _____
23. _____
24. _____
25. _____

SAMPLE BEHAVIORAL ACTIVATION RECORD

Day	Expected time	Activity	Mood before	Mood after
Monday	8:00 A.M.	Going to coffee shop	–3	–1
Tuesday	3:00 P.M.	Bike ride for 30 minutes	–3	–1
Wednesday	7:00 P.M.	Book group	–2	+1
Thursday	12:00 P.M.	Walking dog	–3	–2

In-the-Moment Strategies: How to Keep Depression from Ruining Your Day Once It Hits

If you wake up depressed in the morning, what can you do to keep it from dragging you down, other than just taking medications? Unlike prevention, *harm reduction strategies* are things you can do to reduce the severity or impact of symptoms as they occur.

 "I can't get anything done because I can't get up in the morning. I just want to sleep."

STRATEGY 1: Set a goal for your wake-up time and make it earlier every few days

In severe depressive states, simply being able to get up before noon may be your first challenge. If that is true for you, make that the goal: to be out of bed by noon. If that works, make the next day's goal to be up by 11:45 A.M. A few days later, shift it to 11:30 A.M.

STRATEGY 2: Delay going back to bed in the morning

If you get up, say at 8 A.M., have breakfast, and then go right back to bed by 9 A.M., try to delay going back to bed by 1 hour (10 A.M.) and then gradually delay by 30 minutes each day until you are awake for several hours at a time. After doing this for a couple of weeks you may not need to go back to bed at all. One of the best strategies for depressive states is just staying awake and active for as much of the day and evening as possible.

STRATEGY 3: Take only one nap, at a prescribed time each day, instead of several naps

Try to limit naps to 1 hour or less and make it the same hour every day, instead of many different naps of varying lengths. Try to delay your nap until after lunch, as going back to bed after breakfast can make it more difficult to get going later in the day.

STRATEGY 4: If you are feeling very depressed and lack energy, keep the demands on yourself simple and don't ask too much of yourself at first

Set modest goals, such as getting up by a certain time, putting on your slippers, and making a cup of coffee. The important part is to convince yourself that you're able to keep your morning routine, even if it has become more difficult.

>> Review the more detailed strategies for improving your sleep in Chapter 6.

 "No matter what I want to do, negative thoughts and disaster scenarios get in my way."

Nearly everyone with bipolar depression reports that this state is characterized by cycles of negative thinking and rumination: worrying over physical and emotional symptoms and disaster scenarios (for example, "I feel like I'm going to die") that cause considerable distress. It can be hard to convince yourself that there are alternative ways of thinking, making it hard to move forward with your daily tasks.

STRATEGY 1: Keep a thought record

Keep a simple diary of your negative or pessimistic thoughts, following the structure in the tabular thought record example (page 28), although you may want to modify it for your personal preference. Write down the "automatic thoughts" that occur spontaneously, how they make you feel, and whether you judge the thought to be helpful or unhelpful. Ask "detective questions" about the evidence for or against the thought, and entertain an alternative thought that considers a different angle. This is not the same thing as thinking happy thoughts. It's taking a more scientific approach to your thoughts and evaluating whether they really fit your experiences.

STRATEGY 2: Observe your thoughts from a "decentered" stance

The thought record can feel unrealistic if you're not convinced of your alternative thoughts. Challenging and restructuring thoughts is only one way to deal with negative cognitions. You can also "invite them in." Imagine they are no different from the rumblings of your stomach. Observe the negative thoughts one by one and accept that they're present without chasing them away, but not necessarily buying into them either. Try doing this during a meditation session (see Prevention Strategy 2, Try Mindful Meditation, on pages 22–23).

 "My mind goes round and round in circles, thinking of all the things I've done wrong and the disasters that will follow. I start ruminating about how terrible it is that I'm ruminating. It's an endless cycle."

SAMPLE THOUGHT RECORD

Automatic thoughts	Mood (−3 to +3)	Is this a helpful thought? (Yes/No)	Detective questions *Am I sure this is true? How certain (1–100)? What's the evidence pro/con? Any recent events contradict or support it?*	Alternative thought *Come up with another way to think about this; be more balanced in your predictions.*
"I have no friends."	−2	Unsure	How was it hanging with Susan last week? How often am I busy on the weekends?	"This has been a week of feeling lonely, but I know I have people who care about me."
"I don't feel well so I shouldn't go to work." "I'll do a terrible job if I go."	−1	No	Does staying at home make me feel any better? How often do I do a terrible job at work?	"I'll go for a couple of hours and see how I'm feeling; things are usually better by afternoon."
"Only bad things happen to me." "I can't perform well under stress."	−3	No	I'm focusing on that job interview I ruined, but did I want to work there? When did I last crash when under stress?	"This was a bad break but it's just one job option; I've done much better in other interviews."
"I'm not going to (this party) because no one there will want to hang with me."	−2	No	What happened the last time I went to a party? Were there people I knew, and did they talk to me? Did I meet anyone new?	"It never turns out as badly as I expect; I usually find someone to talk to."
"I'm always going to be depressed and things will never improve."	−3	No	Have I been depressed all the time in the last 6 months? How do I know what will happen in the next 6 months or a year? What new strategies am I using?	"The last time I felt down like this, it took a while to come out of it but my feelings did get better."

STRATEGY 1: Use distraction tools

When you find yourself ruminating (repetitive thinking about negative things, continually worrying about your distress and what caused it, feeling stuck), a simple strategy is to distract your mind:

- Do a puzzle or try to figure out the words to a song.
- Take a moment to notice everything around you and describe it into your phone.
- Sit in a meditative posture and focus on your breathing.
- Stick your hands or your face in ice water. It can be unpleasant and you probably won't look forward to doing it, but it will quickly shift your attention to your physical sensations rather than thoughts.

STRATEGY 2: Set a time limit for ruminating

Set aside 10–30 minutes a day and purposefully ruminate during that time, but only during that time. *Try* to ruminate during that interval. If your mind finds the rumination topic again later, tell it to wait until the next appointed time.

STRATEGY 3: Stop trying to figure out the solution

The problem you're worrying about (say, "I may lose my job") may be important but have no immediate solution. Tell yourself that you don't need to solve the problem right now, that it's OK to refrain from thinking about it outside the time you've allotted to it. Indeed, you are probably not solving the problem by thinking about it.

STRATEGY 4: Reframe the problem

Try to think of the good things about the situation you're ruminating about. For example, if you think you did something wrong at work and will get fired, think of the various good things that might come from getting fired (finding a job that better uses your skills or gives you more satisfaction, for one). Another example: If you're ruminating about the loss of a romantic relationship and whether the other person is dating someone else, imagine that their new partner has rescued you from a potentially destructive relationship.

 "Nothing has really worked for my depression—I'm out of solutions. What else is there?"

STRATEGY: Consider emergency medical treatment

Sometimes depression is so severe that it has to be treated medically. However, the medications traditionally used for depression can take several weeks to take effect. Are there any more rapid alternatives?

STRATEGY A: Ask your doctor about ketamine

If you are really down and have been for weeks, ask your doctor about the anesthetic drug ketamine, which has rapid efficacy for depression and suicidal thinking. Ketamine has been found to quickly lift even very severe bipolar depressive states when other medications have failed. Some studies find that it can alleviate depression in as little as 40 minutes. Ketamine is not provided in every clinic, but it is becoming more commonly available. In the clinic, ketamine is usually administered in an intravenous drip or a nasal spray (esketamine [Spravato]). There are also pill, liquid, and nasal preparations that can be taken at home, depending on your doctor's recommendations.

There are a few caveats. First, the benefits of ketamine are short-lived, about a week to 10 days. It is not a drug you want to self-administer at frequencies higher than prescribed. It is addictive: Some people get into a habit of using the nasal spray every time they feel sad or anxious, which makes it not much better than a cocaine addiction. There are also some worrisome side effects. Some people experience perceptual distortions (such as seeing faces in the trees), dissociation (feelings of unreality or detachment), numbness, or (rarely) hallucinations when taking it. It can temporarily increase your blood pressure and heart rate. Nonetheless, ketamine appears to reverse severe depressions that haven't responded to other treatments, so it is an option worth discussing with your doctor.

STRATEGY B: Opt for transcranial magnetic stimulation (TMS)

Electroconvulsive therapy (ECT or "shock treatment") is still the most effective treatment for people with severe depression who have not responded to other treatments, but it inspires fear in many people. There is now a less invasive technique called TMS. This method involves placing a stimulator coil over your scalp and administering pulses of electrical activity to the dorsolateral prefrontal cortex, which is the major site in the brain for decision making, planning, mental flexibility, and mood regulation. TMS is not as effective as ECT, but it also has fewer side effects and is not as intimidating. There is not much research on this method for bipolar depression (it is FDA approved for major depressive disorder). Additionally, it is expensive and not always covered by insurance.

STRATEGY C: Choose hospitalization for a respite

Hospitalization is necessary when you're feeling suicidal or can no longer take care of yourself. No one looks forward to hospitalization, but sometimes it's the best solution for unremitting depression. What surprises many people is not only the treatments they get in the hospital but also the effects of being away from the daily stressors that elicit low mood states. Hospital stays are a respite, a place where you can get sleep, reestablish a viable daily routine, obtain supportive therapy, and get your medications reevaluated. Sometimes, inpatient physicians will recommend a drug "washout," where you taper off all of your medications and gradually start new ones. This is best done in the hospital given the side effects of stopping or starting new medications.

>> Discuss these options thoroughly with your doctor. If you're not currently depressed but you've been in this state before, it's good to have discussed these options and have plans in place in case it happens again.

Strategies for Talking to Your Family When Depressed

One thing I have consistently heard from people with bipolar depression is that family members usually try to be supportive but don't know what to say or do. They are well-intentioned but say things that feel invalidating or at worst, quite hurtful. If you live with parents, a spouse, or siblings who help you arrange appointments, obtain your medications, provide living space, or offer you financial help, it's important to educate them about what bipolar depression is really like (see the Informational Handout on page 32, an abbreviated description of BD). Their only frame of reference may be their own anxiety and stress, which, unless they have BD themselves, are likely to seem trivial in comparison to your experiences.

Family members can be of considerable help if they understand what you need. My colleagues and I developed *family-focused therapy* (FFT) for this purpose, to help people with BD and their family members gain a shared understanding of BD and learn tools for communicating about matters related to the disorder and family life. Its effects are most powerful in preventing or delaying episodes of depression, but it's also effective in helping stabilize existing mood episodes. This is not surprising; family support is one of the most powerful sources of protection

An Informational Handout for Family Members

Depressive Phases of Bipolar Disorder

Depression in bipolar disorder (BD) comes in episodes that can last anywhere from a couple of weeks to several months. During a depressive episode, I may feel very sad, down, anxious, irritable, numb, or some combination of these. I may have insomnia or sleep too much (with trouble getting up in the morning), lose interest in things, have low energy, move or talk slowly, eat very little (or at other times, too much), feel worthless and hopeless about the future, and have thoughts of taking my own life. Depressive episodes are not like ordinary feelings of sadness. They are much worse and can make it very difficult to accomplish even small things, like taking a shower or getting dressed. I may feel like sleeping the whole day.

Bipolar disorder has a basis in the activity of neural circuits in the brain. Depression is treated with medications, usually mood stabilizers, like lithium or lamotrigine (Lamictal); and sometimes with antipsychotic agents, like quetiapine (Seroquel) or lurasidone (Latuda). It is a good idea for me to have psychotherapy as well, so that I can learn strategies for coping with stress.

I know that I need to take medications, but I also go through periods of doubting whether they help. It won't help me to be constantly reminded to take my medications. Our family may also benefit from seeing a therapist who knows about how BD affects family relationships. What I need most from my family is support in the form of listening when I'm feeling distressed, showing compassion, and, if I ask, helping me communicate with my doctors.

I am still a human being who values my independence, so please respect my wishes in terms of who you contact or consult about my problems. If you are worried about my safety, communicate with me on what you're worried about. Please be patient. Know that I am trying as hard as I can, even though it may look like I'm giving in.

I may benefit from regular daily routines and activities. I may ask your help in coming up with a daily plan to take my mind off my moods. Some of these will be activities that you may want to join me in (for example, going for a hike or doing some deep breathing and meditation). Other things I may want to do alone.

With treatment and family support, I will come out of this. I can accomplish many of my goals for work and family life.

for people who have mood disorders. Here are some of the things you can do to obtain the kind of support from your family that will help most:

STRATEGY 1: Tell your relatives (parents, partner, siblings) what you do and don't want them to do when you are depressed

Your relatives may be "flying blind" in deciding what to say or do when you're depressed, so it can help for you to be clear about what you want. For example, some people find it helpful for their partner to get them up and on their feet in the morning; for others, that would be torturous. Some people find it helpful to have their relatives talk to their medical providers, and others do not. Depending on who is doing it and how, it can feel intrusive or invalidating or supportive and of significant help.

STRATEGY 2: Help them understand why judgments and criticism aren't helpful

If your relatives are being critical or pestering you about your motivation or functioning (such as saying, "You're lazy" or "You need to try harder"), make clear how their judgments are affecting you. You may need to educate them about depression as a biologically based disorder and how different your depressive episodes are from ordinary states of sadness. Consider the informational handout on page 32 as a way to start that education.

STRATEGY 3: Ask your relatives to help you implement a behavioral activation plan

What helps when you feel inert or apathetic? Do you want your relatives to do any of the things on your activities list with you: a walk, some light exercise, going to a coffee shop for an hour? Telling them to "just leave me alone" is telling them what *not* to do, not what you want them to do. Show them your sample behavioral activation record (page 25) so they know what you're trying to do each day and why.

STRATEGY 4: Take turns actively listening

Being able to talk regularly to a validating, accepting person who cares about you—whether a parent, spouse/partner, or friend—can be as powerful as any medication. You may have to make that point clear to your family members. Explain that "I find it most helpful when you just listen and don't try to solve my problems for me." That doesn't mean they can't say anything, but coach them to let you clarify what you've been feeling internally and what roadblocks you've experienced in trying to get through it. Can you talk to them about your recent romantic breakup or job loss? Encourage them to ask questions about what happened and how you're feeling, and coach them to summarize or paraphrase your answers (for example, "So you were really hurt when she said that"). Paraphrasing makes the listener feel that they're not just being passive; they are helping you move forward by understanding what you are distressed about. When it's their turn to share their viewpoint, show that you are listening actively by nodding your head, asking clarifying questions, and paraphrasing what they're feeling. Later in the conversation, when you feel that they get it, you can reward them by encouraging them to voice their suggestions.

>> Review the steps of active listening in Chapter 7.

STRATEGY 5: Reinforce your family members for their efforts

Everybody wants to feel that they've been helpful, so if they've assisted you in getting through an afternoon with less misery, tell them so ("I appreciated your taking that walk with me and hearing about my stuff. It felt good to be heard," or "I know I get irritable sometimes when I'm depressed. I still find your presence to be comforting"). Even if you haven't found them to be helpful, you can still say, "Thanks for being there."

STRATEGY 6: Acknowledge your relatives' demands but assert yourself when the demands seem unrealistic

When depressed, even the simplest request from your family members can feel like a gargantuan task. If your parent or spouse starts making many requests of you and you feel that the requests are unrealistic, nod your head and summarize back to them what they've asked ("I know that you feel strongly that I should be looking for a job"). Then you can add, "I don't know if I can do that right now." They need to know that you've heard them even if you can't follow their advice.

STRATEGY 7: Set limits on questions about taking your medications

Being asked repeatedly whether you've taken your medications is probably irritating, and may make you feel like not taking them at all. Relatives who do this may be genuinely worried about whether you're following your treatment plan, *or* they may not know what else to say or do. Bring the conversation back to the stressful experiences you've had, but avoid getting into a push/pull with them about whether you really have taken all your pills or gotten your blood levels tested. Conversations that go in this direction can be very unrewarding for both parties. Know your own boundaries and be willing to assert them.

Taking Stock

If you have implemented some of these strategies for coping with depression, take stock of what you've learned and what was or wasn't helpful. Ask yourself the questions in the box directly below.

Questions to Assess
a Recent Episode of Depression

- Looking back, what do you think caused your most recent bout of depression? What stressors had a role?

- Were there any early warning signs that told you depression was on its way?

- What medications did you take, and which ones do you think were the most helpful? Consulting your mood chart should help here.

- What behavioral strategies were helpful? Behavioral activation, challenging your thoughts? Mindful acceptance?

- What did your physician and therapist do that was/wasn't helpful?

- What did your family members (or close friends) do that was/wasn't helpful?

2

mania

MINIMIZING SEVERITY
AND REDUCING FREQUENCY

Mania can creep up on you. It can wreak havoc in your life and in those of your family members. You can't fully prevent mania, but you may be able to minimize its severity and frequency. Because it's so difficult to get yourself to seek help when fully manic (described in the box on the facing page), the most effective strategies involve knowing what you've experienced before when headed into mania and making plans to prevent early warning signs (also called *prodromal symptoms*) from escalating into full-blown episodes. But even when you're taking mood-stabilizing medications and doing your best to stay stable, you can cycle into mania. This is certainly not your fault but it's important to take extra measures to minimize harm once in a manic state. What emergency strategies can you implement to keep yourself and others safe?

You may have questions that don't fit neatly into the box. For example, you may want to know "What do I do when I'm depressed? Is that the time to work on preventing my manias?" or "What if I'm already on the upswing—do I still use the same strategies?" This chapter answers these and other questions. It is divided into sections on what you can do (1) when you're stable (or depressed) to prevent future manic episodes, (2) when you're showing early warning signs of mania, and (3) when you're acutely manic to reduce harm. These strategies are summarized in the table on page 38 to give you an idea of the control you can exert at various stages of the manic escalation.

A separate section on hypomania offers similar strategies for episodes that are less severe and do not cause immediate harm. It's important to know how to

Full Episodes of Mania

For most of the time during at least 1 week, mood is "high," or irritable, with extreme expression of emotion and energetic behavior focused on goals. The episode doesn't have to last a week if emergency treatment shortens it. You must be experiencing three or more of the following changes during the manic phase (four if your mood is only irritable):

- Having higher-than-usual self-esteem (such as the belief that you have special powers, are more intelligent than everyone else, or have unique plans for solving important global problems)

- Talking more and rapidly, feeling like you can't stop talking

- When speaking, jumping from one topic to another, or feeling like your thoughts are speeding along

- Sleeping less than usual, or not sleeping at all, without being tired the next day

- Having your attention drawn to unimportant stimuli in your setting, such as background sounds, colors, or traffic noise, making it very difficult to focus; or having trouble distinguishing important from unimportant thoughts or topics

- Feeling physically agitated, driven, and restless

- An increase in impulsive, risky, or dangerous behavior, such as spending money excessively, driving recklessly, or having multiple sex partners

prevent hypomanic episodes because they tend to bring on depressive episodes (or patterns of rapid cycling) when they lift.

The last section of this chapter describes strategies for coaching your family members on ways to communicate their concerns either before or during full manic episodes. As you saw in Chapter 1, there are healthy and unhealthy ways for them to express themselves and equally healthy or unhealthy ways for you to respond.

Strategies for Preventing Full Episodes of Mania

 "When I emerge from mania, I see what I could have done differently, and then I feel ashamed. How can I have better foresight? What will make these symptoms less destructive?"

Preventing Mania and Hypomania and Reducing Harm

Problems I've had during manic or hypomanic episodes	What to do to prevent or minimize the problem when stable	What to do if I'm escalating	Harm reduction when fully manic or hypomanic
I stop sleeping altogether	Keep a regular sleep and wake schedule	Talk to my doctor about medication adjustments to improve sleep (or use previously prescribed sleep agents)	Have a regular bedtime even if I can't sleep; ask my doctor to recommend sleep medications
Drinking or taking drugs that accelerate my mood state (e.g., cocaine)	Avoid all substances of abuse; attend Alcoholics Anonymous or Narcotics Anonymous groups, or see a therapist specializing in substance abuse therapy (such as motivational interviewing)	Decrease access to and contact with drug suppliers; avoid friends with whom I use drugs or drink (see Chapter 12)	Stay away from drugs and alcohol at all costs; enlist help from others in doing so
Going out late at night and having impulsive sexual encounters	Use my support system: nominate a friend/partner to go out with at night, gain their agreement to intercede when I'm in my high periods	Take my friend/partner along when going out at night; avoid places that have led to trouble in the past (such as certain bars or dance clubs)	Challenge overly optimistic thoughts about how wonderful a new sexual encounter will be
Spending lots of money that I don't have	Keep reminders in my wallet about the disadvantages of manic thinking; put a warning sticker on my credit and debit cards	Put spending limits on credit cards or leave them under someone else's control; use 48-hour and two-person decision rules; notify financial broker or bank of need for financial limits	Give up credit and debit cards altogether; pay for things only with cash
Throwing out my prescription pills	Write a list of "Why I should hang on to my medications" that I can access when I want to dump them	Have at least a 2 weeks' supply of my medications in a safe or with a trusted friend	Review "Why I should hang on to my medications" list; talk to my doctor about whether changes in regimen are needed
Getting in my car and driving on highways or long or winding country roads with no speed limits	Nominate someone whose judgment I trust to advise me on driving when my judgment is impaired	Follow their judgment about whether it is safe for me to drive, or take Ubers or other rideshares	Give car keys to trusted person; avoid driving altogether
Other manic or hypomanic behaviors (list):	What I can do to prevent them while stable:	What I can do if I'm starting to escalate:	Harm reduction strategies when manic or hypomanic:

STRATEGY 1: Reality checks for stable periods

Spoiler alert: The high of mania can feel irresistible at first. When you're feeling stable, or even when you're feeling mildly depressed, remind yourself that when you're escalating into mania you may toss aside the habits that have been keeping your moods stable. It is difficult to cut off the escalation because of the following:

- The high feelings are intoxicating, and stopping them is like spoiling a good party
- You don't want to give up your feelings of creativity and productivity
- You're enjoying feelings of power and control

These states are nothing to be ashamed of; they are shared by many people with BD. Yet the measures you take while stable are key to preventing full manic episodes. So, what can you do to give yourself a reality check when enjoying the highs of mania?

STRATEGY 1A: Carry a card in your wallet with warnings

"Sure, this feels great—until it doesn't" and "Power is addictive . . . and it's also an illusion when it comes from mania" are possibilities. Ideally, place the card so that you see it when you take out your driver's license and ATM or credit cards. If you're a frequent user of your ATM card when manic or hypomanic, put a sticker on the back (not near the strip) that says "Not to be used when feeling revved or amped" (or whatever words you'd use to describe your manic or hypomanic state). You may find it equally useful to put these phrases on your phone's desktop.

STRATEGY 1B: Use your support system

Anticipate the kinds of things you've done while in manic phases and think about how others can help you if those occur again. Who in your support system could help keep you from drinking, using illicit drugs, spending excessive amounts of money, or going out at night to places where you could get yourself in trouble? Often this is a friend or a relative who is in your age group and can understand your drive states, even if they have not observed your manic episodes previously.

STRATEGY 1C: Keep healthy sleep habits

You already know about the importance of keeping regular sleep and wake times, habits that are disrupted significantly when mania starts to escalate. Having a predictable bedtime routine (such as, half an hour of reading, a shower, or other relaxing activities before getting in bed) will help you should your sleep patterns inadvertently change (for example, you are assigned a later shift in the workday and decide to stay up later and later to compensate).

>> Review the concrete strategies for battling insomnia in Chapter 6.

STRATEGY 1D: Avoid the daily habit of using alcohol or drugs (or cannabis), even if you think they help balance your mood

Substances of abuse can interfere with the protective effects of mood stabilizers.

>> Review the issues concerning substance abuse in Chapter 12.

STRATEGY 1E: Stay consistent with your medications

As you'll read in Chapter 13, many complex feelings get stirred up in deciding whether to take recommended medications. If you're in the sweet spot of being stable and thinking constructively about the future, that is not the time to go off your medications. Talk to your physician about adjusting your dosages if you are suffering from painful side effects, but stay consistent, using automated reminders (such as watch alarms or notifications on your phone) or pillboxes as needed. Always keep a few weeks of your daily dosages in a safe place, perhaps in someone else's hands so that you don't run out at a key moment in your mood cycle.

When you're feeling well, it is useful to write out a list of "why I should hang on to my medications" that you can access when you feel like throwing them all out. On this list might be considerations such as "I don't want to go through the trouble of renewing and ordering these medications later if I'm in an episode," "The pills have cost _____ dollars and may not be covered by insurance if I try to renew them too quickly," or "I promised _____ (my doctor, spouse, partner) that I wouldn't just throw them away without discussing it with them first."

STRATEGY 2: Create a mania prevention plan

The *mania prevention plan* is an important tool to construct when you're well, using all sources of information available to you (your recollections of prior episodes, diaries, others' recollections, or input from your doctors). Having a prevention plan will give you a greater sense of control over your future. Create your own form like the one shown on the facing page and make sure it lists the following:

- Early warning signs of mania
- Stressors that in the past have preceded episodes

MANIA PREVENTION PLAN

Early warning signs	Stressors or triggers	Coping skills	Troubleshooting	Workarounds

- Potential coping strategies to slow things down
- Identifying and troubleshooting factors that interfere with your coping strategies
- Workarounds for minimizing interferences

If well constructed, the plan will allow you to enjoy some of the benefits of mild hypomania (feeling 'buzzed' or more creative but not out of control) without having to suffer its more deleterious consequences. Your family members or close friends are key allies in developing this plan. So is your doctor, as you'll see below.

STRATEGY 2A: Be aware of your early warning signs

If you're feeling stable now, or perhaps on the mild side of depression, consider the last time you were manic or hypomanic. Scan through your history (or your mood chart or journals if you kept them), make a list of the first signs that told you that you were speeding up, and put these in the first column. Typical are increases in the speed of your thinking, including feeling smarter than everyone else; feeling full of life, joy, or energy; not needing as much sleep; being easily irritated or annoyed, especially by how slowly everything and everybody moves around you; and a boost in your desire to consume material goods, food, alcohol, sex, or drugs. These impulses usually build over a couple of weeks, but the length of the early phase (the prodrome) varies considerably from person to person. Some people say it's a day or two, and others say it can last several months.

If you are always a bit hypomanic by nature, it may be harder to notice these changes. That's how the observations of family members (along with ratings on your mood chart) can help. They may not be familiar with these warning signs unless you have educated them about BD (see Chapter 1) or they were around during your prior episodes. Keep in mind that they will be processing your symptoms from a different observational vantage point, one that places more emphasis on your external behavior and less on your internal experiences. If you ask them what they would put on your list of warning signs, they may say, "You were full of yourself" or "You were incredibly angry at us." Even if you don't recollect those attributes (or perhaps feel that you had ample reason to be irritated), add them to your list of possible early warning signs.

STRATEGY 2B: Identify your stress triggers

Cast your memory back to the environmental circumstances in which your last episode of mania or hypomania occurred. Episodes can be triggered by one's environmental stressors, as well as genetic predispositions and biology. Knowing what stressors affect you the most can help you assess when you are most at risk for a new episode. For example, one person with BD became manic whenever the new university semester began. She developed a plan with her doctor to increase her lithium during the first few months of school while she was adjusting to a new sleep schedule. Events that cause a change in your sleep/wake cycles are potent triggers of mania (starting a new job, taking a plane to a different time zone), but other stressors can play a role as well: new romantic relationships or breakups; "goal attainment" events that involve major accomplishments or opportunities, especially if they involve large sums of money; and severe family conflict or discord.

In the second column, list stressors that you think may have been associated with at least one prior episode. There need not be a direct relationship between the stressor and specific early warning signs, or you may be uncertain which came first ("I flew to Europe on impulse, lost a night of sleep, and couldn't sleep the next night but didn't feel tired"). Nonetheless, identifying the role of stress in the escalation into mania will make you more alert when similar stressors happen in the future.

STRATEGY 2C: Inventory your coping skills

In the third column, list skills you've used in previous manic episodes (or skills you believe you've acquired since then) that could be implemented when the first alarm bells go off. For example, imagine you are needing less and less sleep (and don't feel tired) and have been taking on multiple new projects. Here are some things you can do:

• Keep the times you go to bed and get out of bed regulated from night to night, even if you have trouble falling asleep. Be aware of going to bed (or falling asleep) way later than usual.

• Talk to your doctor about whether changes in your medication regimen are needed. For example, if you are taking an SGA, they may recommend a higher dose when you feel yourself racing. These prescriptions can be written before you develop early warning signs, with the agreement that you'll be in touch with your doctor when you start taking the revised dosages.

• This is not the time to stop your medications. People often stop taking mood stabilizers or antipsychotics and get manic shortly thereafter. It also happens the other way: people start getting manic and then stop their medications because they feel so good.

• If you've had trouble with spending in the past, protect your money. For example, hand over your credit cards to a trusted person. Allow yourself access to an ATM card only with an expressed daily limit of $200 or less. Be especially aware of large purchases involving musical instruments, cars, jewelry, and pieces of art, which, when you're getting manic, may seem like fantastic ideas. See also the discussion below of the 48-hour and the two-person rule for delaying decisions.

- If you regularly invest in the stock market and work with a broker, you may want to let them know that you are prone to overspending when manic or hypomanic, with instructions not to allow you to invest over a certain amount. This is one of those things that you may be able to do when first ramping up but will no longer seem reasonable to you when you're manic.

- If you've had trouble with auto speeding, limit your access to vehicles when you are starting to feel elevated—ideally, give your car keys to someone else.

- Hypersexuality is a common sign of escalating mania. Avoid going out at night alone, especially if you are prone to impulsive sexual encounters. Take a trusted friend or family member (preferably an age-mate) along.

- Be especially cognizant of your intake of alcohol and street drugs, which tend to be overconsumed as one approaches mania (often to chase the high and accentuate it).

- Avoid or at least delay making major life decisions about jobs, marriage, or moving.

STRATEGY 2D: Reduce the obstacles to using your coping skills

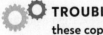 **TROUBLESHOOTING:** "What could interfere with using these coping skills?"

WORKAROUND: List potential workarounds to block these interferences

You may have tried some of these strategies before. In the second to last column, list the factors that have interfered with your attempts to slow down your escalation. Then, in the last column, describe how you might use workarounds. Here are a few examples:

 TROUBLESHOOTING: "I don't even know when I'm getting manic. It all happens so fast. How do I slow it down?"

WORKAROUND 1: Look at the previous 2 weeks of your mood chart and see if there were any "bumps" (short high periods) of a day or two

Many people say that their manic episodes come on almost overnight, too fast to have done anything about, but when they look systematically at the previous few weeks they discover warning signs. This is where having kept a mood chart for several weeks will help.

WORKAROUND 2: *Think about warning signs that occur in combination*

It can be difficult to tell what is a warning sign or what is just a temporary change in mood or sleep that anyone would have. Getting irritable once is not necessarily a warning sign but getting irritable at several different people over a 2-day period and also having trouble sleeping may indicate a heightened risk for mania. Spending a lot of money over a weekend may be just a fun-filled shopping spree, but substantially overspending when you are experiencing an elevation in mood is a red flag.

 TROUBLESHOOTING: "Great idea to call my doctor, but I can't ever reach him. He's never there when I need him. How can I deal with this?"

WORKAROUND 1: *Get a prescription you can use when you're experiencing early signs of mania*

Rather than frantically trying to call your doctor's office when things are out of control, you can develop a reasonable medication plan in advance for when you first notice warning signs. For example, your physician may write a prescription for a new antipsychotic to be taken if you are sleeping less than 5 hours/night or feel agitated and driven. Alternatively they may recommend a higher dose of your mood stabilizer. You can fill the prescription when you're well and have it at the ready when you start to escalate.

WORKAROUND 2: *Call your doctor's backup specialist if your doctor is unavailable*

Discuss with your doctor how you can get help from the doctor who is covering on days or nights when they are away.

 TROUBLESHOOTING: "When I start getting manic, I want to do what I want to do now. How do I slow myself down?"

WORKAROUND 1: *Use the 48-hour and two-person rule*

When manic, people want to do things on impulse and don't want to hear from others that they can't do it. If you want to make a sudden major life change (like marrying someone you've just met or investing a great deal of money in one thing), wait 48 hours before carrying out the decision *and* consult two people you know well (preferably at least one family member) about whether they think it's a good idea. If they dissuade you, you may feel angry and still want to do it, but some part of you will question the wisdom of the decision. Delaying impulse-driven decisions, especially when you have some doubts, is usually a good strategy.

Refer to the table Preventing Mania and Hypomania and Reducing Harm on page 38 for additional workarounds for problems you may have experienced during prior manic episodes. Add in other examples and workable strategies based on your own experience.

Harm Reduction: Strategies for Damage Control When You Do Become Manic

? "I hate the chaos caused when I become manic and my family scrambles around to get me help. What can I do to minimize that?"

STRATEGY: Use emergency and hospital services as necessary

STRATEGY A: Call your psychiatrist and ask for an emergency evaluation

Your doctor will probably recommend either an increased dosage of your mood stabilizer or adding/increasing the dose of your antipsychotic. They will not recommend an antidepressant at this stage.

STRATEGY B: Consider inpatient treatment

Having a manic episode may require going to the hospital, an alternative that will be unwelcome when you're in the midst of an episode. It's best for you and your family members to develop a hospitalization plan when you're feeling well. Make a list of the specifics of which hospital to go to, where the emergency room is, your insurance information, phone numbers of your doctor(s) and therapist, and, although it may not be necessary, contact information for the local psychiatric emergency team.

Of course, the whole purpose of the prevention strategies in this chapter is to avoid hospitalization, but sometimes it's necessary despite your and everyone else's best efforts. You will feel resentment at giving up your independence for this period of time, but keep in mind that you will gain it back later, when you're stable.

STRATEGY C: Be sure your trusted relatives know to inform your doctor/therapist if you end up going to the emergency room or hospital

All too often, people go to the hospital and their doctors only find out after the fact, when it's too late for them to be of help. They should be conversing with the health care workers who work in the emergency department and inpatient unit so that medications that have previously been ineffective or intolerable are not recommended.

Dealing with Hypomania

 "I have bipolar II and only get hypomanic—it's not that severe but it can be pretty upsetting anyway. Is there anything I can do to reduce the damage?"

Hypomania is the same thing as mania except that the symptoms generally do not last as long and are not as severe or disruptive to your life. When people get hypomanic, they may sleep 4 hours per night instead of 7. They may have many creative ideas (of uncertain feasibility) and increase their activity level (such as exercising to excess) in manifold ways. They may try to juggle multiple romantic relationships or spend money extravagantly, but they will not end up in jail or in the hospital. Hypomanic episodes may or may not represent a danger to you, but they do have a way of bringing on depressive episodes in their wake. So, preventing hypomania may also prevent a subsequent depressive (or mixed) episode.

PREVENTION STRATEGY 1: Use some of the prevention tips above but in less extreme form

Don't go driving long distances by yourself, keep your credit cards but be aware of your tendency to spend impulsively, and avoid shops where you've spent money in the past.

PREVENTION STRATEGY 2: If you're prone to calling people at all hours, ask your partner to hold on to your phone for you after a certain hour

If you are not with a partner and don't want to give your phone to your parents, siblings, or roommate, consider shutting it off after 9:00 P.M.

PREVENTION STRATEGY 3: Ask your physician to describe strategies for managing sleep during hypomania

They may describe behavioral strategies for insomnia (see Chapter 6), such as structuring your bedtime routine, or they may recommend a medication for sleep. Usually sleep agents are prescribed on a time-limited basis (such as during the week or weeks of escalation into mania) and generally are taken as needed, not every night. The choice of sleep agents includes the sedative trazodone; Belsomra or Dayvigo, which are dual orexin receptor antagonists; or benzodiazepines like alprazolam (Xanax) or lorazepam (Ativan). Alternatively, they may prescribe a low-dose antipsychotic such as quetiapine (Seroquel) on a time-limited basis. Seroquel is sedating and may cause cognitive dulling the next day, so discuss the pros and cons of each option with your doctor.

Strategies for Talking to Your Family When Manic or Hypomanic

As we saw in Chapter 1, communication with your family will take a hit when you cycle into mood episodes. Your relatives are important sources of input, but when escalating into mania or hypomania you won't want to hear cautions or advice from anyone, least of all your family members. You may hear their suggestions ("You'd really better see your doctor") as reflecting their desires to control you, when the likelihood is that they are feeling scared or confused, with thoughts like "I'm afraid you'll get hurt" or "I don't really know what else to say." Here are a few workaround conversations:

 "I can't listen to what my family tells me when I'm ramping up. How can I hear them without feeling like I'm giving everything up for them?"

STRATEGY 1: When you're well, role-play with your relatives how they might communicate with you when you're becoming manic

When your mood is stable and it feels comfortable, role-play an exchange with your spouse/partner or another family member where (1) you play yourself in an escalating manic state, and (2) they experiment with different ways of expressing their concern about you such that you can hear it. For example, if they say, "You're getting manic and need to get on your medications quick," ask them to rehearse saying, "I'm concerned that you'll hurt yourself or someone else, that you won't be safe. How can I help?" Another example: If they say, "You have to see your doctor; I'm making an appointment for you," ask them to rehearse saying, "It might be a good idea for us both to go see Dr. _____ and make sure we're all on the same page."

It will be easier to pull these responses from your memory banks if you've rehearsed them when you're feeling well. Your natural tendency might be to fight your family members, but when you're well you can practice more reasoned replies: "I know you want to help, but I need to make the decision myself to see my doctor," or "I'll let you know if I've decided to stop taking my meds—I know that's important to you."

STRATEGY 2: Choose a family spokesperson

When escalating into mania, family interactions may go better when you interact with a particular relative with whom you've felt trust during previous episodes. That might be a parent or a spouse or a sibling, but it could also be a more distant relative (like an aunt or uncle) or even someone outside the family. When the family has concerns, they can convey them to that person instead of communicating with you when you're already feeling resentful. Of course, when mania takes hold, you may not want to talk to that point person either, but you may feel differently about them talking with your psychiatrist, in which case you should sign release-of-information forms in advance.

>> Choose one family member or friend to serve as the family's point person. Your doctor will appreciate having one person to contact rather than several people calling them with different concerns.

Taking Stock

The table on page 38 summarizes the prevention strategies we've covered. Use this table as a reference when you're well, when you're experiencing early warning signs, or even when you're manic or hypomanic and feel like things are getting out of control. There are spaces below the table to list other behaviors that have caused you trouble in past episodes and ways you might be able to prevent those from occurring in the future.

These strategies should help you avoid manic or hypomanic episodes or at least reduce their severity, frequency, or duration. Nonetheless, our brains and bodies are on their own trajectory. If you've gone through a cycle of escalation or a full manic episode despite trying these strategies, review your prevention plan and make some revisions. Ask yourself the following:

- What worked about the plan and what didn't?
- Were there things that happened (including what people said) that made you decide to go off of your medications?
- How could the environment have been more accommodating? When would you have been most likely to hear your parents' or spouse's advice? Did they offer "too little, too late"? Were there work or school requirements that kept you up late?
- Would you have been more likely to respond if someone outside the family had expressed their concerns about you?
- How could your doctor have been more helpful, or your therapist? Be willing to discuss it with them.

If you have succeeded in staving off a manic episode, congratulate yourself (and if appropriate, your relatives): You have accomplished one of the hardest tasks as a person with BD.

3

coping with anxiety and worry

Anxiety is a feeling in the body that gets translated into worry and apprehension in the brain. In people with BD, it can occur for long periods of time, seemingly on its own trajectory. Alternatively, it can occur during depressive, manic, hypomanic, or mixed states. Severe anxiety is usually experienced as a strong feeling of nervousness ("butterflies"), excessive worry or ruminative thinking (perseverating on certain thoughts over and over), a feeling of lack of control over events about to happen, and wanting to run away. According to one person with BD type II, severe anxiety is "the most god-awful feeling I've ever had."

Anxiety is a bit like a car alarm—sometimes it will sound because someone is breaking into your car, and at other times for a nonevent, like the wind blowing or leaves falling from a tree. Part of the challenge in dealing with anxiety is determining when the alarm is legitimate.

Consider what happens when people experience "anxious arousal" or panic. Often, panic is generated spontaneously, frequently in a crowded place (like a packed grocery store) or in places where escape is difficult (in a highway traffic jam). When in one of these situations (the trigger), your heart will beat faster, your breathing will speed up, and you will feel a growing sense of unease or apprehension. Some people interpret these bodily sensations as normal reactions to a crowded place, whereas others think it signifies a heart attack and impending doom.

What happens next is most important. If you choose to wait out the physical sensations, you will start to "habituate" and the anxious arousal will drop on its own, as shown in the diagram at the bottom of this page. If you choose to run from the situation (such as pulling your car over at the next exit and parking), your anxiety level will probably drop quickly and you'll experience a sense of relief, but in the long run you're contributing to your anxiety. Eventually you'll have to get back on the highway.

You might decide later that you don't want to drive on that particular highway (can you tell that I live in Los Angeles?) or at that time of day. If panic happens again on a different highway, you may decide you don't want to drive at all on major highways. Your world has just gotten a bit smaller. Yet, had you just stayed in the car, eventually your anxious arousal would have dissipated on its own. Most behavioral treatments for anxiety prescribe doing just that—exposing yourself to the feared situation, experiencing the physical sensations of anxiety and arousal without escape or avoidance, and learning that the sensations go away on their own. Unfortunately, it can be hard to predict how long the anxiety will last, which is why many people choose the escape or avoidance route.

How common are problems with anxiety in BD? By some estimates, as many as 75% of people with BD have had one or more anxiety disorders too, meaning recurrent panic attacks, generalized and impairing worry, social anxiety, posttraumatic stress, or obsessions and compulsions, with significant day-to-day impairment. Some doctors view anxiety as just a part of manic or depressive episodes.

THE VICIOUS CYCLE OF ESCAPE AND AVOIDANCE

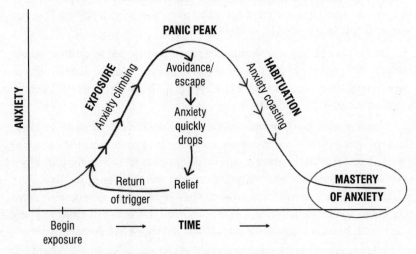

From *Worried No More: Help and Hope for Anxious Children* by Aureen P. Wagner. Copyright © 2002 Lighthouse Press. Reprinted by permission.

Those practitioners emphasize getting your mood symptoms stabilized (usually with medications) before treating your anxiety. However, not everyone with BD finds that anxiety disappears when their depressive or manic/mixed episodes are over. Other practitioners believe that anxiety can be targeted separately from mood episodes, even if implementing behavioral strategies can be harder when you're depressed. I'm in this camp.

Strategies for Preventing Anxiety from Arising

Preventing anxiety states is best accomplished with a combination of monitoring yourself and cognitive-behavioral *exposure strategies*. There is also a role for medications in preventing anxiety.

STRATEGY 1: Track your anxiety in relation to your mood changes

As you did for depression and mania, you can track anxiety symptoms using the mood chart, simply by using the right side of the chart to rate your daily anxiety level. Use a 1–5 scale to show how anxiety fluctuates with your depression or mania symptoms. A rating of 1 is the most calm you've ever felt (maybe on a vacation, lying on the beach), and 5 is the most anxious state you can imagine (panicking in a public place, feeling unable to breathe, losing control of yourself, and sobbing). There are many gradations in between, but try to rate your average for the day. Rate your physiological arousal level, not whether you have had a stressful day with lots of work or have had to deal with traffic jams; those are contributors to anxiety but not the state itself. Rate your anxiety level while reading this: Are you feeling anxious at an average level for you (such as a 3)? More relaxed than usual but not the most relaxed you can be (2)? Very anxious, with heart palpitations, shallow breathing, or sweating (5)?

Once you've made anxiety and mood ratings together over several weeks or months, certain patterns will start to emerge: anxiety heralds the onset of depressive, manic, or mixed episodes by a few days; anxiety always occurs along with depression (in which case it probably will clear when your depression lifts); or anxiety stays around at a severe or impairing level even once your depression or manic or mixed symptoms have stabilized (in which case it may be a separate condition that requires treatment of its own).

There are features of anxiety that distinguish it from depression. Depression is usually about past events, whereas anxiety is usually worry and perceived threat regarding current or future events. When you have thoughts such as "This is not going to work out well," or "I'm going to be humiliated," you are thinking in the future tense. Other symptoms of anxiety include heart racing or palpitations, sweating, agitation, and gastrointestinal symptoms. Depression is usually experienced as deep sadness, loss of interests, insomnia, and low energy. Some symptoms overlap, such as feelings of restlessness or changes in appetite.

STRATEGY 2: Use the anxiety reduction plan to track situations, cognitions, and behaviors

Tracking your anxiety or worry levels has a more immediate goal: to increase your awareness of how anxiety, mood, thoughts, and behaviors are connected. For example, you may have anxious ruminations that precede the start of the work-week ("How am I going to get that spreadsheet together before the Zoom call?"), which may then lead to avoidance of certain work tasks, which then leads to falling behind at work. Recognizing these patterns can be the first step in altering them. On the back of your mood chart, or perhaps using a notes or spreadsheet app on your phone, create an anxiety reduction plan like the one on the facing page.

The anxiety reduction plan starts with identifying the times or situations where your anxiety level has reliably increased, such as being in crowded places, in settings where you are expected to speak to strangers, or where you feel threatened or judged harshly. For now, just record these situations in the first column and how anxious each makes you feel in the second column. If your anxiety is always present regardless of the situation (as is true for many people), record the situations that stand out as provoking more anxiety than usual. Later, we'll record behavioral and cognitive coping strategies and roles for your family members in reducing your distress. I have filled out the first two lines as examples.

STRATEGY 3: Use cognitive-behavioral treatments

A key element of your anxiety reduction plan is engaging in regular cognitive-behavioral therapy (CBT), preferably with an individual or group therapist but also by implementing strategies on your own. Discuss with your prescribing physician—or with your therapist if you have one—whether you could benefit from one of the CBT programs summarized in the table on page 56. After reading over the descriptions, ask whether the doctor knows of clinicians who practice these treatments in your area. If you are fortunate enough to already have a therapist who provides one of these treatments, you won't have to arrange treatment with many different providers.

SAMPLE ANXIETY REDUCTION PLAN

Situation	Anxiety level (1–100)	Things I thought or predicted	How much I believed the thought (1 = not at all, 3 = some, 5 = completely)	Alternative thoughts	Behavioral strategies used (e.g., deep breathing, meditation, distraction)	Anxiety level afterward (1–100)
Being in a supermarket	70	"I'm going to have a panic attack."	4	"I've been here many times before without panicking."	Sitting down, deep breathing, distracting myself	40
Talking to my teacher/ professor about a grade	50	"She'll think I'm stupid and I'll feel humiliated."	3	"My questions aren't worse than anyone else's; this teacher seems nonjudgmental."	Standing up, taking deep breaths, being aware of my thoughts	30

A Brief Guide to Cognitive-Behavioral Therapy for Anxiety

Treatment	For what?	Description	Where to go for more information
Cognitive-behavioral therapy	Generalized anxiety and worry; social anxiety	Cognitive restructuring, relaxation, exposure to worrying thoughts, tolerating distress states, and problem solving; mindfulness and relaxation exercises; exposure through behavioral assignments (e.g., conversations with strangers)	*https://div12.org/treatment/cognitive-and-behavioral-therapies-for-generalized-anxiety-disorder* *www.medicalnewstoday.com/articles/cbt-for-anxiety#_noHeaderPrefixedContent* *https://nationalsocialanxietycenter.com/cognitive-behavioral-therapy/social-anxiety-strategies* see also *www.toastmasters.org*
Cognitive processing therapy	Posttraumatic stress disorder (PTSD)	Focuses on cognitions about traumatic events, why they occurred, and how to reinterpret them	*https://cptforptsd.com*
Exposure therapy	PTSD and other anxiety disorders	Uses a variety of techniques (in vivo, imaginal, virtual reality) to expose you to feared stimuli in a safe environment, to reduce fear and avoidance	*www.apa.org/ptsd-guideline/patients-and-families/exposure-therapy*
Exposure and response prevention	Obsessive–compulsive disorder and PTSD	Exposes you to stimuli (such as dirt or germs) that generate obsessions and make you want to perform rituals (such as hand washing); treatment teaches you to not perform compulsive behaviors and to use alternative coping strategies	*https://iocdf.org/about-ocd/ocd-treatment/erp*
Eye movement desensitization and reprocessing (EMDR)	PTSD	Combines exposure techniques with eye movements to reduce the vividness of trauma memories	*www.emdria.org/find-an-emdr-therapist*
Panic control treatment	Panic attacks	Education, cognitive restructuring, relaxation, controlled breathing procedures, and controlled exposure to physical sensations that contribute to panic	*www.nimh.nih.gov/health/publications/panic-disorder-when-fear-overwhelms*

Finding therapists who practice these interventions is not always easy, but there are a number of mobile apps that enable you to try these techniques on your own (the MindShift CBT app is one: *https://apps.apple.com/ca/app/mindshift-cbt-anxiety-relief/id634684825*). Generally, though, mobile health apps require at least some contact with a therapist or behavioral coach to be effective.

The treatments described in the brief guide to CBT (page 56) have all been found to be effective in randomized controlled trials with people who have anxiety disorders. Behavioral treatments rely on *skills* as their primary tools for managing anxiety (such as gradually exposing yourself to feared situations or focused exposure on your internal thoughts or sensations), as well as the techniques with which you're already familiar, such as cognitive restructuring (challenging negative beliefs and rehearsing alternative and more adaptive thoughts). The skills described in the guide can be listed in your anxiety reduction plan.

STRATEGY 4: Talk yourself through anxiety-provoking situations

If you regularly become anxious in certain situations, and you are going to be entering one soon, imagine entering the situation and write a script about your behavior in it. For example, imagine you have a terrible fear of going to the dentist. Write out your worst-case scenario. Here is an example:

> "I park in the parking lot, and the attendant gives me a dirty look. I arrive at the office and am told I have to wait 15 minutes. I imagine myself perspiring and wondering if anyone can smell my perspiration. I know I'm going to panic once I'm in there, like start to hyperventilate or maybe do something awful, like pee on myself or throw up. The dental hygienist will be disgusted by me, and I'll end up running out of the office."

Notice how many negative, disaster cognitions occur in this mini-essay and how many of them involve being publicly embarrassed or physically aversive to others. Very little of the imagery has to do with having one's teeth cleaned or getting hurt by a dental instrument. This is where "detective questions" come in handy: What is the evidence that any of these things will occur? Will everyone (or, really, anyone) be able to tell you are anxious, and why would that make them disgusted by you? Have you ever peed on yourself or run out of the door? What is the likelihood (on a scale of 0–100%) that any of these things will happen? And if you are sweaty or breathe a little heavier when you go to the dentist, is that really so unusual? Don't other people get anxious at the dentist's office? What thoughts will help you feel OK with that possibility?

Next, rewrite the scenario such that you use some of the anxiety-reduction techniques you're already learning in this chapter:

> "I park in the parking lot and, even though the attendant is unfriendly, I smile at him. Before I go into the office, I sit on a bench and do a few minutes of deep breathing, becoming aware of my body and breath. I enter the office and continue to meditate while I'm waiting. Once I'm inside, I rehearse thoughts like "I can do this," "I've handled this before and it doesn't matter if people think I'm anxious; lots of people are anxious when they go to the dentist."

If you can identify a particular stimulus in this sequence that triggers you (like the parking attendant's look or the smell of dental hygiene products), try a sitting meditation before going, in which you casually scroll through your memories of those stimuli and "invite them in." Imagine yourself having coffee with the parking attendant or purposefully smelling the dental products as if they were perfumes. Whenever you find yourself getting anxious, pay attention to the feelings in your body. You can always return your attention to your in-and-out breathing if this becomes difficult.

STRATEGY 5: Take the pharmacological route

Sometimes the behavioral treatments above are combined with medications. Discuss with your doctor whether antidepressant medications would be advised to prevent major bouts of anxiety or to manage impairing levels of worry and apprehension. Antidepressants within the SSRI class (see Chapter 1; for example, escitalopram or Lexapro, sertraline or Zoloft) are often recommended for anxiety. These carry a risk of mania or rapid cycling, but if they are accompanied by an adequate dosage of a mood stabilizer or an SGA, they will probably be safe and possibly effective for preventing and managing anxiety states.

Antidepressants can take between 4 and 8 weeks to show their full effects, so they are not to be taken on an as-needed basis. If you go this route, you have to give them a fair chance: 2 months is usually long enough to determine their benefits, although this length varies depending on whether you are also in a mood episode.

In-the-Moment Strategies for Anxiety

 "How do I cope with all these worrying thoughts and disaster scenarios?"

For most people, anxiety is an immediate problem, one that haunts daily life. Fortunately there are things you can do while anxiety is building or once it's already present. Imagine you are out and about (for example, sitting in a movie theater) and start experiencing growing signs of distress, even if you can't pinpoint their origin. What can you do?

STRATEGY 1: Adjust your breathing

Fast and shallow breathing is associated with "fight-or-flight" states, whereas slower, deeper breathing is associated with relaxation. Sit in your chair and relax, using one or more of the following methods:

STRATEGY 1A: Slow it down

At rest, your breathing should be 12–20 breaths per minute, but with focus you may be able to slow it to seven or eight, with longer gaps in between. The slower you breathe, the more you will feel a sense of calm.

STRATEGY 1B: Try 4–4–8 breathing

Breathe in for a count of 4 seconds, hold your breath in for a count of 4 seconds, and then exhale for 8 seconds. Keep doing this—with intervals in between—until you feel sufficiently calm. None of these techniques is specifically designed for BD, but they take advantage of the relationship between breathing and our body's stress response system.

STRATEGY 2: Remind yourself of constructive thoughts in the moment

Imagine you are entering a challenging situation and are already feeling excessively anxious about it (say, a job interview). First, prior to the interview, write down your thoughts ("I'm really going to come across as weird in this job interview") on your anxiety reduction plan (page 55) and mark how strongly you believe in them (1 = *not at all*, 3 = *somewhat*, 5 = *completely*). Then, ask yourself, "Is this thought useful? Is it going to help me?" Ask yourself some of the detective questions illustrated above: "What is the evidence that I won't be able to handle myself? Why would this person think I'm weird?" Generate some alternative thoughts and write these on your plan as well: "Everyone feels nervous at job interviews," "I've come across well in the past," and "This isn't a make-or-break situation." Note whether your thoughts are self-defeating or involve "negative forecasting" ("If this happens again, my life will be ruined") and introduce some alternative thoughts for those as well ("No one event is ever going to ruin my life").

Anxious thoughts tend to be the most potent in situations in which you are being evaluated in some way. Rehearsing alternative thoughts will not immediately calm you in the moment, but they will likely temper how much anxiety you feel and help put others' evaluations in context. In moments of anxiety or stress, remind yourself of these alternative thoughts by reviewing your anxiety reduction plan or by keeping a record of them on your phone. Some people find it helpful to summarize them with a memorable line or mantra ("Move toward, not away, from things that scare you").

STRATEGY 3: Use a meditative technique for negative thoughts

As you learned in Chapter 1, an alternative to challenging your thoughts is to focus on them, experience the strong emotions they generate, and accept these thoughts and feelings as part of yourself. They will lose their potency the longer you observe them, much like exposure exercises decrease the potency of the situations you fear. It's best to do this when you can carve out some time:

- Try sitting in a meditative pose (usually in a chair with your eyes closed). Let your mind wander and focus on your breathing.
- As negative thoughts appear, imagine them like playing cards pulled one by one out of a deck (for example, "there's the card about relationships . . . there's the one about money . . . here's the Jack of job interviews). Concentrate on the thoughts for a few minutes, even if you find them disturbing. This helps you get some distance from them, taking a nonjudgmental, observing stance.
- When you feel anxiety start to rise, avoid trying to chase it away. Instead, be aware of it and experience it fully.
- If the anxiety becomes intolerable, gently move your attention back to your breathing or other sensations in your body.

STRATEGY 4: Consider anxiety-reducing medications

In-the-moment anxiety can also be brought under control with benzodiazepines, like Xanax (alprazolam) or Klonopin (clonazepam). Doctors are reluctant to prescribe benzodiazepines because there is a high addictive potential. There are other options, such as hydroxyzine (Atarax, Vistaril), which is an antihistamine for allergies that has sedating qualities; or gabapentin, an antiseizure medication also recommended for anxiety. None of these medications work immediately; benzodiazepines, for example, generally take at least 30 minutes to kick in fully.

If you anticipate your anxiety becoming extreme in certain situations, that may be the time to take a benzodiazepine (or gabapentin, or hydroxyzine, depending on what you've been prescribed). Taking anxiety medications won't cure your anxiety-inducing thoughts but they will reduce your level of physical distress. Just be cognizant of how frequently you use these medications: Any antianxiety medication has the potential to become addictive.

Getting Help from Your Family

As was true of depression and mania, family members and friends can be of help or hindrance when you're anxious. Following are some options to discuss with them so that they know how to be helpful. If you find these suggestions effective, include them in a separate column in your anxiety reduction plan. Once again, it's best to have these discussions with your family when you're feeling OK, rather than when you're in the height of anxiety. At those times you may feel resentful of their suggestions, or you may just want to get away from them.

STRATEGY 1: Explain how bipolar anxiety is different from ordinary anxiety

In BD, anxiety is driven in part by biological processes that are not fully under your control. The worst thing that parents or a spouse can do is criticize you or be dismissive of your fears, making you feel like a wimp. So, explain to them: "When I get anxious, there are parts of it that are not under my control, and I need your support. It doesn't help to hear that I'm being stupid, or weak, or a worrywart, or 'just deal with it.'" If they ask you what would help, say, "Just let me express what I'm feeling anxious about, and listen without judgment. You don't actually have to say anything or give me any advice."

STRATEGY 2: Take them along

Gradual exposure to anxiety-producing situations can be aided by having a friend or family member accompany you in those situations. If you've been depressed recently and are anxious about becoming socially active again, it may help to have a sibling, cousin, or close friend go to a social event with you. It can also help to have them join you in everyday tasks that make you anxious. You can say, "I'd like to ask you to do something with me that I ought to be able to do myself: grocery shopping. Having you there as a companion will help a lot." There is no guarantee that they'll say yes, but they will probably feel good that you value their company.

Next, imagine the scenario where your spouse or partner has made social plans—such as a dinner party—but you feel too depressed or anxious to accompany them. You may have known about the plans for months, and may have agreed to them initially, but right now a dinner party feels about as fun as having all your teeth removed. Can you push yourself to go as opposed to giving in to your desire to avoid it? Stay for 30 minutes and then decide whether you want to leave? If you feel this is impossible, then the next best thing is to encourage your spouse to go without you: "I'm not feeling well and I don't want to ruin this event for you. I'd rather you went without me (or with _____ [friend])." Your spouse or partner will feel less resentment if they are able to proceed on their own without feeling like they're abandoning you.

STRATEGY 3: Tell family members to avoid "accommodation"

There is a more subtle way that family members can unwittingly contribute to your anxiety: by accommodating it. *Accommodation* refers to encouraging your avoidance behavior or even amplifying it. For example, imagine that you are prone to reassurance seeking ("Can you remind me if I turned off the stove?"). A family member who is accommodating will offer repeated reassurances, even though you don't really need them. This behavior tends to be most common in obsessive–compulsive disorder, where family members decide to help you complete cleaning, washing, or checking rituals just because it seems more efficient than waiting for you to do so.

Explain to your family members that accommodating may alleviate your distress in the short run but it won't help in the long run. For example, you may feel like asking them to go back in the apartment or house and check to make sure the stove is turned off before you leave for the evening. It's best that they don't do this; they can respond with "I'd rather not get into that." If that feels too harsh at first, advise them to reassure you verbally once but not multiple times. Avoid incorporating them into compulsive rituals, such as watching you wash your hands or being willing to wait an extra half an hour while you take a second shower.

Taking Stock

Implementing these strategies can be very difficult, even though I've made them sound easy. Anxiety is part of the human condition, but it can be especially impairing in BD. Depression amplifies anxiety, and anxiety contributes to low moods.

Go back to your anxiety reduction plan and see if you can fill out some of the columns. What items in the plan are likely to work? If you tried something and it didn't work, what can you do differently next time? Take some time to revise it accordingly, with a focus on these questions:

- If you took antianxiety medications, what was their impact? Have any been effective in the moment? How often did you use them?
- What behavioral strategies have you tried? Have you tried gradual exposure to the situations you're most uncomfortable about? Used meditative or breathing techniques? When have they helped and when not?
- How has challenging your thoughts worked? Were you able to generate alternative thoughts in the moment, or did you get stuck with the same thought over and over again?
- How have family members helped or not? What can you advise them to do differently?

4

dealing with irritability and anger

Being excessively irritable is a common problem for people with BD. It is usually a symptom of depression but can also be a symptom of manic, hypomanic, or mixed episodes. However, some people with BD feel chronically irritable independent of their mood state. The feedback you may get from others takes the form "I have to walk on eggshells around you." In others, irritability is episodic, occurring intensely in some situations or with certain people but not with others. It may be influenced by the context (such as loud restaurants), how many people (or whether certain individuals) are present, or whether alcohol is involved. What distinguishes bipolar irritability from everyday irritability is its intensity and potentially destructive quality.

Being excessively irritable is not your fault. Neuroimaging studies indicate that neural circuits in the brain (specifically, those involving the ventricular prefrontal cortex and the amygdala) may become dysregulated in people with BD when they are in highly emotional situations. If your irritability is interfering with your daily functioning—your ability to complete the workday or school day or relate in a civil way to those you encounter—look to this chapter for recommendations on how to minimize the damage. You may not be able to prevent getting irritable, but you may be able to limit its expression and impact in your daily life.

As was true in earlier chapters, your support system is valuable here. You probably don't want your parent(s), spouse, or close friends to interfere in your conflicts with others, but family members or friends can help you in ways you may not expect, by helping you process what went wrong in confrontational situations. Your closest supporters are probably aware of your irritability and may welcome ways to minimize its impact, particularly when they are on the receiving end. In turn, you may be able to explain to them why certain things they do or say trigger your intensive emotional reactions. In this chapter you'll learn strategies for anticipating and coping with your anger in reaction to the people in your life. Conflicts in family relationships, which are often driven by issues such as your desire for greater independence; violations of your confidentiality or trust; or, more generally, feeling like you are being treated like a patient rather than a son, daughter, sibling, or partner, are the subject of Chapter 7.

Preventing Aggressive Outbursts

 "I'm constantly pissed off. How can I control this?"

Have family members or others been complaining that you're irritable "all the time"? Just hearing that may make you feel irritable, especially if you think it's an unfair or exaggerated characterization. Nonetheless, if you're worried that your irritable outbursts are alienating others in your life, the first strategy for prevention is to determine whether you really have been as irritable as others claim. Most of the preventive measures that follow involve using the information you gather after the day's events to determine what you might do to dial down irritability and minimize its impact on your quality of life.

STRATEGY 1: Track your irritability or anger outbursts for 2 weeks

Keeping track of your irritability may help you determine how severe it is and whether it has been going on for too long. There are many ways to chart your irritability. The simplest way is to make a single 1–5 rating each day of how irritable, angry, or bitter you felt and how much of a problem it posed for you (also on a 1–5 scale). If your mood and irritability are highly variable, make one rating at the beginning of the day and another at the end. For example, you might rate the morning a 2 and the afternoon a 1 if you had one brief negative exchange with your spouse or kids before work, but otherwise your irritability didn't cause any problems. Try doing this for 2 weeks and determine if it stays high, varies with the time of day, and how much it interfered with your daily life.

A potentially more informative way of tracking irritability is to add it to your mood chart. You can add a line for anger and track it alongside of your depression or mania symptoms and changes in sleep patterns. You can add notes on the chart with details on the situations that evoked your anger. Knowing whether high irritation happens when you're with certain people or when you haven't slept well the night before can help you prevent irritability from hijacking what you want to accomplish that day. You may even discover more subtle patterns, such as anger episodes that are elicited by situations where others seem to be questioning your stability.

In the example in the chart on the facing page, Roxie modified the left-side mood words to distinguish "energized" from "superhyper" and "down" from "depressed." Her anger/irritability (the dashed line) was fairly constant throughout the week, but it got worse when her depression (solid line) worsened on Wednesday, when she argued with her boyfriend. For Roxie, this pattern suggested that she was (at least in part) communicating her depression to others through anger, or perhaps that her anger led to an altercation, which made her feel depressed.

Irritability is often triggered by certain interpersonal situations. Common triggers for people with BD are interactions with people in positions of authority, such as teachers, bosses, police, or religious figures. Parents usually occupy positions of authority and are common targets of anger outbursts; so are spouses or partners, especially when power differences in the relationship start to feel imbalanced. In your chart, you can characterize the target of your anger with codes such as F (with family member) or B (boss); whether the interaction is with a stranger or someone you know (S or not-S); or whether a significant other (SO; a spouse or partner) was involved. When you've collected a couple of weeks of irritability ratings, examine whether they vary with your up-and-down mood swings, how many hours of sleep you had each night, and the regularity of your bedtime and wake time (notice that in the example above, Roxie had the least hours of sleep in the interval between Tuesday night and Wednesday morning). Try also to determine whether certain people or situations are most likely to provoke your anger.

STRATEGY 2: Find out whether your doctor is treating your irritability directly

If you are chronically irritable, you may be undertreated, meaning that your medication dosages may not be high enough (or your medications may be the wrong ones) to control your mood symptoms. Be sure to talk to your physician if you feel your anger is getting out of control and you don't think your medications are doing their job. Your psychiatrist may already have prescribed medications that control

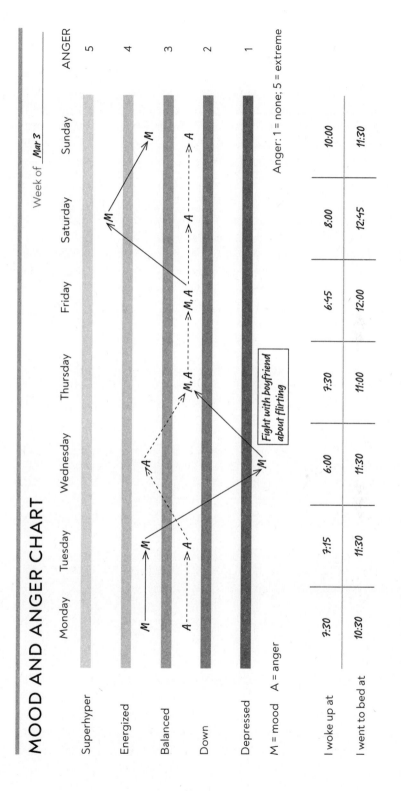

MOOD AND ANGER CHART

Week of _Mar 3_

	Monday	Tuesday	Wednesday	Thursday	Friday	Saturday	Sunday	ANGER
Superhyper								5
Energized							M	4
Balanced	M →	M	→A	M, A	→M, A	M		3
Down	A →	→A		→A	→A			2
Depressed			M					1

M = mood   A = anger

Fight with boyfriend about flirting

Anger: 1 = none; 5 = extreme

	Monday	Tuesday	Wednesday	Thursday	Friday	Saturday	Sunday
I woke up at	7:30	7:15	6:00	7:30	6:45	8:00	10:00
I went to bed at	10:30	11:30	11:30	11:00	12:00	12:45	11:30

irritability and temper outbursts. SGAs like risperidone (Risperdal), quetiapine (Seroquel), or aripiprazole (Abilify) are often recommended when people report periods of irritability that interfere with their functioning. Antidepressants (such as fluoxetine [Prozac] or duloxetine [Cymbalta]) may also serve this purpose. Recall that antidepressants are often used for the control of anxiety as well as depression, and irritability can reflect underlying states of anxiety and lack of control.

Mood stabilizers, antidepressants, and antipsychotics are not meant to control irritability in the moment. They will not work fast enough when taken that way, and you may get the wrong dosage if you are already taking one of these and then take an additional dose. Some doctors recommend hydroxyzine (an antihistamine with a calming effect) or a benzodiazepine like Xanax for harm reduction in situations that readily evoke irritability (like large family gatherings, waiting in long lines). Again, you'd have to take them at least 30 minutes in advance of the event to have any effect.

STRATEGY 3: Be aware of your irritability early in the day

STRATEGY 3A: Pay attention to certain physiological symptoms when you get up in the morning

There are subtle warning signs in advance of getting angry or enraged, such as having violent imagery or "feeling the heat rising." On certain days you may notice that you feel unusually frustrated by ordinary morning rituals (such as not finding your toothbrush) or unduly irritated by your dog or cat. If you have a roommate, you may snap at them first thing in the morning. Your irritability could be justified or due to many factors other than your illness, including the other person's habits or behavior. You may also be hungry ("hangry"), have slept poorly the night before, have had an unresolved argument with someone, or simply may not want to talk or deal with other demands of the day. All of these reactions, of course, are part of being human and may be independent of your BD, but they will be worsened if you are already depressed, manic/hypomanic, or in a mixed state.

STRATEGY 3B: When the day's schedule includes high-risk situations, consider canceling or rearranging them

If you wake up irritable, review your plans for the day and see if any anger-provoking situations can be avoided. If you had planned to have a highly emotional discussion with your partner or a family member, consider having it on another day. If you need to do some shopping at a place that you find frustrating or where parking is an impossibility, put it off, or at least minimize contact with others while in the store by going at the least busy time of day. Make an active effort to reduce your contact with people who readily provoke you, including family members. See the "Taking Stock" section at the end of this chapter for any information you've gathered that identifies these individuals.

STRATEGY 3C: When you can't avoid high-risk situations, use "arousal dampening" through a brief meditation in the morning

If you need to go to work or school anyway—whether that means taking a bus across town or simply telecommuting from your bedroom—you can calm your body and mind by doing a brief meditation, such as a 3-minute breathing exercise (see the box on page 70).

STRATEGY 4: Take a mindfulness app with you

If you begin the day feeling irritable and you need to be away from home for most of the day, keep a brief mindfulness meditation on your phone and call it up before you interact with others. You never know when you might have to go into a highly stressful interaction with a coworker or a stranger, and the more you can do to take control of your reactions, the better these are likely to go. There may also be situations that routinely upset you (such as getting on the subway or standing in a lunch line). You'll find examples of guided meditations that you can download from the app store and take with you at *http://franticworld.com/mindfulness-apps*.

In-the-Moment Strategies to Use When You Get Angry

Consider the following situation. You've been mildly depressed in the last week and also feel more reactive than usual to minor slights. You have to go to the grocery store to get a refund for an unwanted item. Your savings are getting low, and this return feels very important to you. Once there, you're told to talk to the store manager. You know that you're entering a potentially high-conflict situation and that your irritation could escalate into full-blown anger.

STRATEGY 1: Revise your self-talk

Whether it's interacting with a store manager or any other hot-button situation, try to determine in the moments beforehand whether you're overfocusing on issues such as feeling weak or taken advantage of, believing that others think you're dumb or incompetent, or worrying that you'll be dismissed because of the way

3-Minute Breathing Exercise

This exercise will give you a brief experience of mindfulness—being aware of your body, breathing, and thoughts or feelings in the present moment, without self-judgment. You can do this alone or with someone else, but avoid any conversation during the exercise.

Sit in a comfortable chair and close your eyes (or if you prefer, stare at an object in the room), with your back upright and your hands on your thighs, or lie on your back if you prefer. Spend 60 seconds being aware of the present moment. Ask yourself, "What am I experiencing in my mind and body right now? What are my thoughts and feelings? Where in my body am I experiencing tension?" Pay attention to any pleasant or unpleasant feelings or sensations and accept that they are present—there is no need to judge them or chase them away.

For the next 60 seconds, pay attention to the physical sensations of breathing, or simply count the number of times you breathe. If your eyes are open, watch the up-and-down movements of your stomach or chest. Think of your in-breaths and out-breaths as like riding a wave. If your mind wanders, notice what took you away, and then gently return to focusing on your breathing. It's important not to judge yourself for being distracted—the in-and-out movements of your chest will help you stay anchored in the present.

In the last 60 seconds, expand your focus to different areas of your body. Be aware of your posture, your facial expression, and any tension you feel in your feet, legs, thighs, buttocks, stomach, arms, chest, shoulders, neck, and head. Notice what happens in your body as you breathe in and out. Once again, it's inevitable that your mind will wander, but gently escort yourself back to awareness of your body and breathing. When you notice sensations of distress or discomfort, anchor your breath to those sensations and breathe into them and out of them. You may want to tell yourself, "Whatever these feelings are, I'm going to experience them and allow them in."

Last, gradually open your eyes and come back into contact with the room. This exercise will probably relax you and may promote a feeling of acceptance of yourself and others, even if only for an hour or two.

From *The Mindful Way through Depression* (pages 183–184) by Mark Williams, John Teasdale, Zindel Segal, and Jon Kabat-Zinn. Copyright © 2007 The Guilford Press. Adapted by permission.

you look. These are common types of self-talk when one is depressed and irritable. Next, think of some counterthoughts before entering the situation. Examples are "This may be an issue for me (such as how much I weigh) but I have no reason to think it's an issue for this other person," or "I'll do my best to state my case but this person may not have much control over resolution of the problem."

STRATEGY 2: Beware of aggressive nonverbal communication

Early in the interaction with the other person, take a deep breath and listen to how your voice might sound. If your speech is clipped, harsh, loud, or very rapid, you may get immediate defensive reactions from the other person. Avoid raising your voice or talking over them. Avoid standing too close to the person or making jerky bodily movements.

STRATEGY 3: Find alternatives to inflammatory language

Avoid starting sentences with "You did this," or "You pissed me off." Use an "I" statement before making a "you" statement: "I" statements are harder to argue with because they usually indicate that you are "owning" how you felt. In cases like getting a refund, it may not even be necessary to acknowledge your emotional state. Consider the difference between "You never gave me a refund and I'm really annoyed" and "I'd like to know what I can do to get the refund process going."

If you find yourself making accusations or threats, substitute strategies such as paraphrasing what they say before making your side of the argument ("I understand that your policy is not to exchange an item that is 2 days old, but my situation is different because this item was already open when I bought it"). When you make a request, start by taking a deep breath and give the person time to respond rather than jumping in with multiple staccato demands.

STRATEGY 4: Know when it's time to quit, at least for now

If you're getting nowhere, ask if there is someone else you can talk with. Whether or not you get what you want, be prepared to walk away and regroup. You may want to take this up later with someone else, but for now you've done your part.

How Did It Go?

Let's now think about how to put these lessons to work in prevention planning for the next social situation in which you feel irritated. Imagine that you've just had a negative interaction with the store manager. How do you feel about how you handled it? Perhaps you were able to regulate your expression of anger, and if so, well done. Alternatively, perhaps you got angrier than you had planned. Examine your thoughts. Self-talk such as "I should have said . . . ," or "I can't believe what an _____ that guy was" tells you that your irritability may have gotten the better of you.

If you're disappointed in how you dealt with the incident, try to avoid being overly self-critical. You're practicing emotion regulation strategies that are difficult for anyone, bipolar or not. Instead, review *how* the event got you angry and *when*. Try to recall when in the conversation your thoughts turned defensive or when you started believing that you were being treated unfairly.

How Can You Make It Go Better Next Time?

STRATEGY 1: Try compassion meditations

If you want to take mindfulness meditation to another level, try an exercise focused on *compassion*. Compassion requires stepping out of your negative feelings about a person and generating feelings of empathy for them. Once you have calmed down a bit, sit by yourself, perhaps in your parked car or on a bench outside, and observe your anger at a physical level (such as the pounding of your heart or the rapidity of your breathing). Picture the person who just made you angry, acknowledge your irritation, but then imagine wishing them well for the future. In the grocery store example, think about the manager as a fellow member of the human race, one who may have their own problems or be unhappy themselves. This is difficult to do when you're angry, so if you're too upset immediately after the interaction, wait a few hours and try again. Examples of compassion or "befriending" exercises are at *www.youtube.com/watch?v=pLt-E4YNVHU* and *www.youtube.com/watch?v=9JRQMBHjnT8*.

STRATEGY 2: Make some repairs

If you feel you overreacted and expect to interact with this person again, consider using *repair strategies* (see below) to make amends. We will talk more about repair strategies in relation to arguments with your family members, but for now, consider seeking the person out when you're feeling calmer and saying, "I'm sorry I got so angry before. I was feeling a bit rushed and I probably overreacted. Next time I'll try to be more patient."

STRATEGY 3: Use an anger chart for specific events

Do a "postmortem" on the anger-eliciting event using a chart like the one on page 74. This involves recording, in separate columns, (1) your level of irritability before the anger-provoking event (such as 2 on a scale of 1 to 5), (2) what actually happened (briefly, what you said and they said), (3) what thoughts you had (such as "This person wants to take advantage of me"), (4) how the event affected your irritation level ("My anger got to a 5"), (5) how you responded to the person verbally (or physically), and (6) where in this sequence you could have intervened to change the outcome (what else you could have done). Things to think about include: Was this the best time to go shopping? Did I interpret the interaction in the only way it could have been interpreted? If there were other ways to think about it, write those down as cognitions to rehearse the next time (for example, "The guy looked harried and stressed out; it was a Sunday afternoon when that store is always crowded").

Have this chart available on your phone or tablet to record the results of confrontations like this one throughout the day. There will always be unpleasant people and unpleasant situations, and when your mood is unstable you'll be prone to strong reactions. With regular use of these emotion regulation tools, you will feel more and more in control of your interactions with others.

 ### "How do I manage my irritability at work?"

Being constantly irritable in the workplace or school environment is very common for people with BD and presents special issues. Some people with BD decide not to go to work or school on days when they feel irritated. Others disclose their disorder to individuals in their human resources (HR) department (who will invariably inform the employer) so that they can ask for special accommodations (such as starting the workday later in the morning, working in rooms where they'll be less distracted by others, or having more frequent breaks). But as discussed in detail in Chapter 9, there are risks to disclosing your disorder in the workplace, such as having your behavior interpreted in terms of your diagnosis or being fired for reasons that sound like mental health discrimination.

STRATEGY 1: Coping with triggers in the workplace

If you're repeatedly triggered by others in your workplace, consider whether you're in the right job. People with BD can do very well in high-energy, high-stimulation jobs, unless they get easily provoked by obnoxious customers or fellow employees. If you find yourself in a job where you react strongly to customers who treat you dismissively, or a boss who constantly looks over your shoulder, you may be working in the wrong place. Here's an example:

SAMPLE ANGER CHART FOR SPECIFIC EVENTS

Irritability before event (1–5)	What happened?	Thoughts about event	Irritability or anger after event (1–5)	How I responded	What I could have done differently	Other ways to think about the event
Mild, 2/5	Confrontation with store manager over refund	"He's trying to take advantage of me." "He thinks I'm a pushover."	Angry, 4/5	Cursed, stormed out	Waited, took deep breaths, asked to talk to someone else	"The store is understaffed; their refund policy isn't about me."

Melissa, age 21, had bipolar II disorder and was currently in a mixed (depression with hypomania) state. Her job in a music store required that she buy and sell used stereo and musical equipment. Customers frequently arrived without appointments, with large amplifiers, speakers, or instruments that they wanted to dump quickly, collect their money, and go. She had to test the equipment to make sure it worked before the store could buy it. Customers frequently became rude, telling her that she didn't understand audio equipment, that she was cheating them, or that they knew the store would dust off the items and sell them at twice the price. After a particularly grueling day, Melissa blew up at a customer who had made a sexist comment; then she railed at her supervisor before storming out. She spent the rest of the day at home, in bed. Although the store valued her and wanted to have her back, she decided there were more accidents waiting to happen and decided to look for a different job. The job itself, she felt, was becoming a trigger for her mood swings.

If you begin the day feeling irritable, and especially if you've felt this way for several days running, a break from work may be a good idea. Calling in sick or asking for a mental health day is not unreasonable, unless you do it right in the middle of an important project with a deadline, or ask repeatedly for days at a time. Extended breaks from work are best negotiated with your employer, sometimes with the aid of a doctor's note. I have written many such notes for my patients, and they are usually effective in getting breaks or accommodations (such as a change in work hours).

STRATEGY 2: Learn effective problem solving and communication with coworkers

Let's say you're going through a period of hypomania with irritability and you've decided to tough it out at work. You feel that people at work are moving very slowly; you want things now, but become annoyed because your requests are seemingly being ignored. You may be prone to impulsive reactions, such as suddenly getting angry or cursing loudly. If you expect to have a confrontation with a coworker (say, because they have ignored your requests, or they have an annoying habit such as playing their music loudly in the next cubicle and you can't concentrate), apply some of the same strategies that were suggested in the section on conflict with strangers (pages 69–70). Avoid aggressive nonverbal behavior or using inflammatory language; be aware of your physical state and cognitions ("I'm already fuming and this is not going to go well") before approaching the person. Once again, a brief mindfulness meditation may help.

If you know the person well, start with a "joining" statement that acknowledges a shared interest ("I know we're both into hip-hop, and I like your selections, but I'm finding it hard to get my work done because I can't concentrate. Can you turn it down a bit or use headphones?"). Always have a solution in mind—something you want to ask them to do rather than not do. It's often useful to add how it would make you feel if you could resolve this ("I really value our working relationship and I want us to get along").

When evaluating the incident later, consider the work context. Is this a situation that is likely to repeat itself, and is there a broader solution, such as asking the employer to institute workplace rules about playing music, having loud phone conversations, or other distracting behavior? Think about alternative cognitions to rehearse prior to these problem-solving discussions (such as "This is the first time I'm bringing this up—it may not get resolved right away"). If the conversation with a coworker doesn't go well, consider whether repair strategies might be in order (such as saying, "I imagine that conversation felt hurtful to you. I know it's hard to be on the receiving end of that kind of irritation"). With these plans in mind, you are in a much stronger position for dealing with similar conflicts in the future.

Communicating with Family Members about Irritability

> "When I'm depressed and around my family, I have this really bitter, all-consuming anger. I can't even pin it on anything, just this sense of fury for things they said a long time ago or things they did that now seem so minor."
> —*32-year-old woman with bipolar I disorder*

If you're living with a spouse, parent(s), and/or siblings, they are probably acutely aware of when your irritability is escalating. In Chapter 7 I talk in more detail about how to navigate family relationships, but for now, consider whether their knowledge of your emotional states can be used productively. How might they help you cope with emotional reactivity, either with them or when you are heading into high-stress situations with people outside the family?

STRATEGY 1: Help your family members put your irritability in context

If you're noticing certain telltale signs of your irritability early in the day (perhaps you're snapping at family members or cursing more frequently; they tell you that you seem grouchy [or they use more colorful language]), alert them as to why you feel distressed. Does it have to do with them, or something you're doing later that day? Alternatively, you may have noticed an uptick in your energy levels or worsening symptoms of depression in the last week. If you feel comfortable doing so, explain that you're experiencing a return of mood symptoms and that they should try not to "overreact to my overreactivity."

Alternatively, recent interactions with family members may be the main drivers of your irritability. Perhaps they've been hypervigilant to minor changes in your mood or have been bugging you about your medications. Perhaps you've explained the run-ins you've had with strangers and they have immediately pinned the blame on you. The key solution here is to give them feedback in a nonconfrontational and nonjudgmental way. Make it clear that you and they are on the same team. For example, if they confront you on being irritable with them, try this type of response:

> "I know I've been more grouchy than usual. Please try not to take it personally. It has to do with my mood cycles. I'm trying hard not to lash out, but I'm not always successful. I'll try to rein myself in but try not to react too strongly to changes in my voice tone or cursing or whatever—it's the way I'm letting off steam."

Depending on their age and your relationship with them, you may want to go for a walk or a drive with them to talk through whatever situation you're upset about. If you feel that there is too much tension to have a productive conversation, redirect the discussion away from your illness to more neutral topics. Ask them how things are going in their life so that the focus is not always on you. Alternatively, be prepared to walk away rather than engage in an unproductive discussion.

STRATEGY 2: Role-play potentially conflictual interactions

There are other ways your family can support you. Consider the situation where you're going into a work or school situation where the potential for conflict is high. You can tell from your level of irritability that the interaction may not go well. One thing you can do is ask them to role-play the expected interchange with you. For example, in the foregoing example involving a grocery store manager, ask your spouse or sibling to play the "rigid store manager with rules to follow" while you rehearse asking for a refund. Ask them to alert you if your voice sounds clipped or harsh, or if you've cut them off. Alternatively, you can play the store manager while your relative plays you. This has the dual advantage that you may experience empathy for the store manager while also learning of a different way to ask for a refund. Of course, this is only one example, and it depends on your and your relative's being open to doing a role play. Nonetheless, having practiced your role in an upcoming confrontation can help you regulate your emotions when it actually occurs.

Finally, if you come back from having had a negative interaction with someone outside the family, ask them to help you make sense of it without placing blame. Take them through the "I said/they said" of the interaction and try to keep them focused on what was actually communicated by all involved parties, rather than generalizations or criticisms (such as "Well, we know how you get when you don't get your way"). They may have useful suggestions for next time, or perhaps they'll express some empathy for you that you didn't realize they felt.

Taking Stock

We're all human beings, and it can be quite difficult to feel constantly irritable or hostile, even if you know it's part of your disorder or has a biological basis. Your anger may be generated by real provocations, even if it's amplified by your disorder. If adding an anger rating to your mood chart has been useful, make it a regular part of your mood-tracking routine. As you've seen, irritability can be a sign of depression or anxiety or a warning sign of oncoming mania, one that may necessitate implementing the prevention plans discussed in Chapter 2.

Your family members are often walking a thin line between wanting to be helpful and being angry or defensive themselves. They may be wondering why they are in the firing line. When you're feeling better, try some of the repair strategies described above. Show a willingness to collaborate, such as "I want us to have a good and respectful relationship even when things aren't going well. How can we avoid this kind of argument in the future?"

Your family members may insist that you go see your doctor to get your medications reevaluated. Whether to do so is up to you. You will have more "fate control" if you bring these issues up with your doctors directly rather than family members intervening on your behalf. Of course, medication adjustments are not always the answer. Sessions with a therapist in which you explore the triggers for your anger, along with implementing your own coping strategies for managing anger, may be just as helpful.

5

protecting yourself from suicidality and self-harm

Suicide is the hardest part of BD for people to talk about. It still carries a significant stigma for much of society, as if it indicated a weakness or personal failure (or, for family members, failure as a parent, spouse, or sibling). Yet suicidal thoughts and actions are a part of human living and can't be hidden or wished away. The first piece of advice I can offer about suicidal thoughts is to remember that they're an expected part of having BD, and having the thought is not the same thing as acting on it. For some, suicidal ideation has been there all along, even when they're well. For others, it is a symptom of a depressive, mixed, or manic episode. Both forms carry risk and deserve support and treatment.

When you've been through multiple episodes of depression or mania and the traumatic events that accompany them—for example, becoming estranged from a spouse or losing one's job—your confidence gets chipped away little by little, until you can only see yourself as bad or defective. When you add in the stigmatizing and shaming ways that our society discusses mental illness and suicide, and the religious and political beliefs that color these discussions, the risk of self-harm goes up even further.

Nonetheless, suicide is about choices. For some people, suicide is a desire to escape intense and persistent pain. For others, it has "altruistic" motives, with thoughts like "People would be better off if I weren't here." Often absent in suicidal states is the belief that one has options. In this chapter, I explain what you and others can do to prevent self-harm and suicide attempts when you're in the midst of an active suicidal state. Among the most powerful are in-the-moment coping strategies, such as Marsha Linehan's *distress tolerance* tools from dialectical behavior therapy (*https://dbt.tools/distress_tolerance/index.php*).

You can also enlist the support of your family. They may insist that you get evaluated for inpatient care (see the box on the facing page on the criteria used for hospitalization, as well as the discussion of the protective effects of inpatient care in Chapter 1), but there are other things they can do to be helpful, as explained later in this chapter.

Finally, you can read Chapter 12, which is devoted to the abuse of drugs and alcohol. Substance and alcohol abuse are highly relevant to suicidal acts because they decrease your inhibitions against self-harm and aggravate the desire to punish yourself. It is important to understand the complex, bidirectional associations between substance abuse and mood.

Self-Harm Prevention Strategies

There is a lot of confusion about self-harm (such as cutting oneself): Is it just an expression of distress with no real wish to die, as is often claimed? In fact, there is considerable evidence that self-injury increases the risk of actually taking one's life, so it's important to educate yourself and others about the nature of self-harm. You can find such information online (for example, *www.nationalelfservice.net/mental-health/self-harm/harm-reduction-self-harm*). A number of websites and mobile apps, such as *www.mind.org.uk/information-support/types-of-mental-health-problems/self-harm/helping-yourself-now*, can remind you of behavioral options you can use if you feel like harming yourself. No website or app, though, can substitute for getting a full evaluation and treatment from a mental health professional, preferably from someone who understands BD.

What might make you vulnerable to urges to harm yourself? The key factor is usually a feeling of self-hatred, often brought on by a rejection event like a breakup with a partner, public humiliation, or bullying. Social media is awash in stories about depressed teens who begin self-cutting or even make serious suicide attempts after being bullied or shamed, at school or online. In adults with BD, the urge to cut, burn, or otherwise hurt oneself can often be attributed to depressive episodes, although even then there are social triggers that bring about the desire to self-harm.

People who feel the urge to harm themselves aren't always aware of how this

When Is Hospitalization Necessary for Self-Harm or Suicidality?

If you're having suicidal thoughts that are getting more frequent or intrusive (such as popping into your head when you're working or reading or watching TV), or you've already made an attempt or made concrete plans to do so, it is necessary for your family or a close friend to take you to a hospital. You and your family members or friends may disagree on when an inpatient stay is necessary—you may feel you have mentioned suicidal thoughts only in passing, and that they're overreacting. Nonetheless, they may not feel that they can keep you safe and you may not be sure you can do so either. Err on the side of getting an evaluation in the hospital's emergency room (ER). If nothing else, the ER will be an important source of information about treatment options.

The hospital you go to probably depends on your locale, what your insurance covers, or where your doctor recommends. In most hospitals, a doctor and/or nurse interviews you in the ER to determine whether your suicidal thoughts or plans are serious enough to warrant a hospital stay. Although your family members will have input, it is not really up to them whether you're admitted. You should be truthful with the personnel in the ER about your level of suicidal intent, whether you have a plan, and your history of mood episodes and suicide attempts. The criteria the facility will use include whether you:

- Recently made a suicidal attempt or "gesture," such as cutting yourself, taking a large number of pills, or writing a suicide note

- Have stated the desire to die, with concrete plans for how to do so and when

- Have the means to hurt or kill yourself by a specific method (such as using guns, knives, or pills)

- Have expressed significant emotional pain and hopelessness, believing that your mood and situation will never get better and that suicide seems like your only option

Depending on the results of this safety assessment, they may admit you or send you home, hopefully with recommendations for outpatient treatment. They may recommend an intermediate solution like a partial hospital or intensive outpatient program. They may make suggestions on what you and your family members can do before you are next seen on an outpatient basis, although hospitals vary considerably in how thorough they are in their discharge recommendations.

As an adult, it is your decision whether to be admitted or not. The exception is when the doctor believes it is unsafe for you to go home and admits you for observation on a 72-hour hold. The hold enables the medical staff to obtain more information and hopefully allows you some time to decompress and get away from the situations that are eliciting your suicidal thoughts. If you have a psychiatrist and therapist, make sure they know you are in the hospital or ER. Sign release-of-information forms so that the inpatient staff can contact them to share information.

desire overtakes them. But if you experience this urge, it might be because the instinctive desire to preserve your body goes underground when you feel ashamed of and terrible about yourself. Cutting yourself can feel deserved, and it provides a temporary escape from negative emotions (anxiety, sadness, anger) while introducing feelings of peace or even hopefulness. This is part of the reason the behavior persists, even though you know it's bad for you. The cycle continues because the self-harm temporarily pulls you back to reality, but only for a short while as the negative feelings soon return, accompanied by the desire to hurt yourself again. Although it's not easy to do, you can anticipate the sequence that leads to self-harming and intervene with alternative thoughts or behaviors, particularly with the help of a therapist but even by yourself.

 "How do I stop hurting myself?"

In the strategies described below, you'll notice the importance of considering the timing of events in the sequence leading up to self-injury. These strategies should apply no matter how old you are, even though the case example is a person in her early 20s.

STRATEGY 1: Conduct a chain analysis on your most recent instance of self-injury

The chain analysis is a key technique in dialectical behavior therapy, an intervention in which people learn to use behavioral and cognitive skills for emotion regulation, mindfulness, tolerating states of distress, and functioning effectively in the interpersonal realm. If you have been hurting yourself over the previous week, take a day or evening when you feel OK and take the event apart, event by event and thought by thought, taking into account what happened before as well as after the event. When written down, a chain analysis looks like the events described in the box on the facing page.

Notice how Zoe weaves together events, thoughts, feelings, and behaviors in sequential order. It can be hard to do that with self-injury, because the events can seem foggy in retrospect. So, if you're prone to self-injury and know your basic triggers (arguments with a partner, for example), have a phone at the ready and record your thoughts and feelings as the night progresses.

The chain analysis may suggest points at which you could reevaluate your responses or change your environment. For example, Zoe could have gone to talk with someone else at the party; challenged her thoughts that Evan was talking to another woman because Zoe was fat and ugly; or, when she got home and had the

Example of a Chain Analysis

Zoe, age 22, put together this chain of events, feelings, thoughts, and behaviors about a self-cutting incident that had occurred the previous Saturday after a party. She preferred to assign times to each event.

Before 8 P.M., night of the party: I thought that I looked fat, no matter what I put on. I remember thinking that when Evan (boyfriend) came over to pick me up, he looked at me and seemed disappointed. I immediately said, "Don't worry, I'm not going to wear this blouse," and I went upstairs to change it, while he was yelling, "You look fine! Come on, we're late."

8:30–10:30 P.M.: We were at Emily's party. I had a beer and I was feeling drowsy almost immediately because I hadn't eaten dinner. But then Evan saw his ex-girlfriend, Jessie. ☹ She blew me off (even though we used to be friends). She was way more interested in talking to Evan, and it seemed like they were flirting. I felt unattractive, ugly even; the longer they talked, the more I wanted to get out of there and cut myself. I wondered if I could go do it in the bathroom.

10:45 P.M.: I told Evan I wasn't feeling well, so he took me home but was all resentful about it. He usually stays the night but instead he muttered something about going home because "well, you're sick and stuff." Then I started wondering if he was gonna go back to the party. When he left, a few minutes later this song came on my Spotify playlist that reminded me of our trip to Alaska and I started crying.

11:30 P.M.: I called Evan even though I knew I shouldn't. He was still in his car and I asked him why—he wouldn't tell me where he was. He seemed irritated that I had called. I asked him point-blank if he'd gone back to the party to see Jessie. He denied it, got annoyed with me, and said that he thought "maybe we should see other people." I immediately started crying when he said that. I felt ashamed that I wasn't handling it well. When he hung up, I texted Stella, my friend who'd been at the party, to see if he had gone back. But she didn't respond.

11:45 P.M.: I felt angry, hating myself and feeling betrayed by Evan and Jessie and even by Stella. That's when I started cutting myself. I did a few cuts on my upper arm, sort of like a tic-tac-toe shape.

12:00 and later: I felt better after I had cut myself, like I was back to being a real person. I called Stella. I got her as she was going to bed. I told her what had happened, and she offered to come over. She's a really good friend. I told her she didn't have to because I was already feeling better because she had shown a lot of understanding. I just needed some sympathy at that moment.

desire to cut, distracted herself through an ice bath, drawing with a marker pen on her wrists, turning on loud music, or any of the other strategies listed in the sections below. For now, think of the chain analysis as the basis for choosing among the coping skills in a "toolbox."

STRATEGY 2: Reduce access to sharps and pills

This may seem obvious, but the less access you have to implements to cut your skin or overdose, the less likely you are to do it. For most adults, blocking all access to knives, scissors, or nail clippers is impractical. Instead, put these items in a place you can access but have to work hard to get to. A garage with a safe, or a cabinet on a shelf that requires a ladder or stool may be adequate. If overdosing is a risk, keep 1 week of your psychiatric medications accessible and the rest of the month's supply in a hard-to-reach place. The point is to make access difficult so that you have time to process what you are about to do, rather than just harming yourself impulsively.

STRATEGY 3: Schedule distracting activities for times when you're more likely to self-injure

Many people self-harm late at night, sometimes after drinking or using drugs, and often after a negative interaction with their romantic partner. If this sequence has occurred more than once on a Saturday night, make sure that the interval after which you see your romantic partner includes some supportive communication with others. You can ask a friend (or a sponsor from a support group) to expect a call from you on Saturday night once you get home; if planned in advance, you may feel less guilty about interrupting their evening. You can reassure them that you aren't expecting therapy from them; you probably just want them to listen and show empathy and understanding.

There are a number of other distracting activities (see below) to consider implementing at these times. The idea is to plan them in advance, rather than trying to recall them for the first time when you're already feeling desperate.

In-the-Moment Strategies for Self-Harm

 "Once I get in that frame of mind I can't let go of it. I feel like cutting is my only option."

STRATEGY 1: Identify thoughts associated with your desire to self-harm

First, identify the thoughts that are going through your head. Common thoughts include "I deserve to be punished," "It's the only thing that distracts me from horrible feelings," "When I cut I feel like a real person," "It gives me a feeling of control," and "It's a way to get revenge on people in my life [partner, parents]." Write down the thoughts and star the ones that seem most likely to provoke self-harm. Use the chain analysis form on pages 86–87.

STRATEGY 2: Introduce an activity that distracts you and shifts your thoughts and attention elsewhere

These "replacement activities" are especially helpful if self-cutting (or other suicidal acts) are in the service of escaping a negative emotional state. Here are a few options:

STRATEGY 2A: Rub a dry-erase marker over those sections of your skin where you previously have cut or burned yourself

Draw a picture of what the cut would look like.

STRATEGY 2B: Use ice water to distract from cutting

Fill up the sink or a large pot with ice water and stick your hands or your face into it for a few seconds. It will be unpleasant and may hurt, but it will also snap your attention back to reality in the same way as self-cutting.

STRATEGY 2C: Change the scene so that you experience different physical sensations

Take a cool shower, ride on an exercise bike for 5 minutes, or take a brisk walk outside. (Some of these options obviously won't be feasible if you live in an area where you can't safely walk at night.)

STRATEGY 2D: Try a sitting meditation, such as a self-compassion exercise

These exercises (*https://self-compassion.org/category/exercises*) combine meditation with thoughts about being kind to yourself. The latter may be especially useful when you're combatting self-criticism (thinking you've made terrible mistakes or deserve punishment). The exercises can provide you with the same compassion you might give a friend who has made mistakes.

CHAIN ANALYSIS RECORD FOR SELF-INJURIOUS BEHAVIOR

Describe the incident involving self-injury that you would like to focus on. What did you do, where, and at what time?

What emotional or physical states may have caused you distress at the time? List all of the factors that might have contributed, even those that seem unrelated to self-harming (such as a poor night of sleep), physical illness symptoms (a sore throat), recent use of alcohol or drugs, being isolated from people, or medication side effects (feeling sluggish or having headaches). Recall any imagery that may have affected you (feeling disturbed by the way your body looks).

Describe all events (in order of time) leading up to the self-injury and the feelings, thoughts, and behaviors that went with each one. What started the chain? Something you did or someone else did? Draw the sequence in panels if you prefer. For each event, describe what you may have thought and how you felt before and after. Example: "It started when I went to class, felt like I was dumb" or "I talked to my parents—I felt guilty and that I've always been a burden to them."

(continued)

Describe in detail the event that occurred immediately before your self-injury. The event may have been an hour before, a day before, or even a week or more before. When that event occurred, what were your thoughts? Feelings?

What happened after the self-injury event? What did you feel after hurting yourself (include any positive [elation, relief] or negative [guilt, shame] emotions that you recall, in any combination)? What did others do immediately after? Did anyone try to get you to a hospital or call your doctor? Did anything positive or negative happen?

STRATEGY 2E: Try journal writing to express your feelings

If you find it difficult to express yourself using the chain analysis form, try free-form writing about the sequence of thoughts, feelings, and behaviors that led to the desire to harm yourself. Write it like a story. If you are describing something that has already happened, have any new feelings or thoughts surfaced since then? How have others responded to you, and did that help or hurt?

STRATEGY 2F: Put together a playlist (in advance), and then when you're getting upset, turn on the music loudly and either sing along with it or dance to it

The type of music you listen to is up to you—whatever works to get you out of the state that leads to self-harm. Some people prefer loud and angry music; others prefer upbeat dance music or any gradation in between.

STRATEGY 3: Address the underlying emotional state

A difficult but potentially more informative strategy is to try to dig into the underlying emotions and understand where they're coming from, rather than trying to distract yourself from them. Journaling will be of considerable help here. When you look at the chain of events leading to self-harm, what emotion dominates? Was it sadness, guilt, anger, or anxiety? If it was anxiety, some of the self-calming activities in the anxiety chapter (Chapter 3) should be of help. If it was shame, consider what made you feel ashamed, and in front of whom specifically? If it was anger, and you're clear who you're angry at (and why), do a compassion meditation focused on them. Again, try to understand the sequence that led to your cutting:

> "I felt rejected by Evan, and that made me feel worthless, and then I felt angry. When I felt angry, that's when I cut myself so that I could express the anger physically. When I had finished, I felt this sense of relief, kind of like if I had yelled and told him off."

Many people who self-harm or become actively suicidal have been traumatized as a child, often with a history of physical or sexual abuse or the sudden loss of a parent. Explore (preferably with a therapist) the role of trauma or loss in relation to your current pattern of self-harm. How are you thinking about this trauma or loss—are you blaming yourself? Have memories of the trauma become more salient because of recent events in your life? Identifying the association between past events and current suicidal thoughts will not make the thoughts go away, but it will help put them in context. If memories or images of the trauma continually emerge, try substituting some of the distraction and replacement activities under Strategy 2 above.

Strategies for Preventing Suicide

 "How do I stop myself from actually making a suicide attempt?"

So far we've talked only about self-harm, which may or may not go along with a wish to die. How do you prevent thinking about or even acting on more serious suicidal plans—for example, self-cutting or overdosing with the intent to die? When you are in a depressed or mixed state, and especially if you are drinking or using drugs, you are at higher risk for acting on suicidal impulses.

STRATEGY 1: Write a suicide prevention plan

The first step is to put together a suicide prevention plan, as shown on pages 90–91. This is best done in collaboration with your therapist or psychiatrist and, if possible, family members. Write your first draft when you're not feeling suicidal. As you saw with previous prevention planning, it's hard to think of alternative behaviors when you're in the thick of it.

STRATEGY 2: Talk to your psychiatrist about antisuicide medications

Consider whether your suicidal impulses are one in a series of depressive symptoms. Do they go along with insomnia, fatigue, loss of appetite, feelings of worthlessness, or loss of interests? If so, your medications are not fully doing their job. Talk to your doctor about changing to or adding a medication with greater antisuicide properties. Lithium has the best record of suicide prevention in BD, with reductions of 54% compared to placebo pills. Antidepressants and SGAs have their place in suicide prevention as well.

STRATEGY 3: Keep a Reasons for Living Inventory

Marsha Linehan, the psychologist who developed dialectical behavior therapy, recommends completing a Reasons for Living Scale when you're feeling well, to remind yourself of the reasons you don't want to kill yourself. The scale can be found at *https://depts.washington.edu/uwbrtc/wp-content/uploads/Reasons-for-Living-Scale-long-form-72-items.pdf*. Items on this list include considerations such as "I have a responsibility and commitment to my family"; "I want to watch my children as they grow"; "I have future plans I am looking forward to carrying out"; "I am afraid of the actual act of killing myself"; "Other people would think

SUICIDE PREVENTION PLAN

1. **List your warning signs of a suicidal episode** (morbid thoughts; plans involving weapons, times, and places; persistently sad and morose mood; social withdrawal; sleep disturbance, fatigue, and loss of energy; guilt or shame; talking to others about death or the afterlife):

2. **Check all the things you can do if you experience one or more of these warning signs:**

   ❑ Get rid of all dangerous weapons

   ❑ Call your psychiatrist or therapist to arrange an emergency appointment

   ❑ Ask for telephone coaching from your doctor(s) or call a suicide hotline (x988 or 800-273-TALK, or the Teen Line at 800-TLC-TEEN [800-852-8336])

   ❑ Implement replacement activities:

       ❑ Meditation

       ❑ Listening to music

       ❑ Ice bath

       ❑ Exercise

       ❑ Rewarding activities involving other people

       ❑ Other (specify) _____

   ❑ Challenge your self-defeating thoughts about current stressors and consider alternative thoughts about the same situations (such as "It's possible that I'll feel differently about this after I've talked to _____").

   ❑ Ask close friends or family members for support

   ❑ Consult religious or spiritual sources that have helped you in the past

   ❑ Review your Reasons for Living Inventory (see page 89)

(continued)

3. Check off the things your doctor and therapist can do:

❑ See you on an emergency basis

❑ Provide a limited amount of telephone coaching

❑ Modify your medication regimen

❑ Arrange hospitalization if necessary

❑ Help you understand what is causing your suicidal thoughts

❑ Assist you with behavioral strategies for handling painful thoughts and feelings

4. Check those things that your family members or close friends can do. For each item checked, list who you most trust with the task:

❑ Listen to you, validate your feelings, offer suggestions

_____

❑ Avoid being critical or judgmental _____

❑ Distract you with mutually enjoyable activities _____

❑ Help you take care of responsibilities that have been difficult (like child care, cleaning, or taking care of pets) _____

❑ Stay with you until you feel safe _____

❑ Call your doctor or therapist to help arrange an appointment

_____

❑ Take you to the hospital _____

❑ Take away weapons, pills, or other sources of danger to you

_____

5. List your doctors' names and phone numbers:

_____   _____

_____   _____

_____   _____

I am weak and selfish"; and "No matter how bad I feel, I know it will not last." The instructions call for rating each of these items on a scale of 1 (*not at all*) to 6 (*extremely*) of importance. When you have suicidal urges, it may help to pull out the list and remind yourself of the reasons you want to stay alive.

STRATEGY 4: Construct a hope kit

A hope kit or chest contains items that have given you comfort, remind you of close relationships, or symbolize meaning in your life. These can include pictures of loved ones, close friends, or pets; lists of songs you love; souvenirs of childhood (such as baseball cards); favorite perfumes; or even reminders of items from the Reasons for Living Scale, written on individual cards. Then, when you feel depressed or have suicidal thoughts, pull out the chest to give yourself a temporary feeling of comfort and remind yourself that you are capable of being happy.

Getting Support from Your Family

Our loved ones should be the first at our side when we feel suicidal. Unfortunately, many family members (parents, spouse/partner, siblings) do not know what to do when you express suicidal intent or engage in self-harm. Most want to be supportive and show compassion, but how they go about it can feel quite off the mark. The first consideration, then, is to think about how your family members currently react to your suicidal thoughts or acts and whether those reactions have been helpful. If they are not, what would you want them to do or say differently? Many family members say they are much clearer on what not to do than what to do. If you have never told them about your suicidal thoughts, think about doing so and pair the disclosure with suggestions on how they can help.

STRATEGY 1: When you're feeling OK, explain to your relatives how self-harm is a coping mechanism

When I talk to family members of people with BD, I encourage them to understand that a relative who self-harms is suffering and in considerable distress, and using the only coping strategy they know; they are not being manipulative. I acknowledge that this is very difficult to understand from a family member's perspective, especially one who has never dealt with a mood disorder.

Explain to your family members or significant others how self-harm is a coping mechanism for you: "Cutting myself makes me feel at peace, or more real, or more in touch with my body than at any other time. I know it's not healthy and it's not good coping, but at those moments it's the only thing I can imagine doing that would bring me relief."

STRATEGY 2: Explain the causes of your distress

Family members may be more helpful if you can tell them, in a general way, what issues are causing you the most pain. In fact, talking about suicidality with a family member may help you clarify the issues for yourself. Are you feeling suicidal over a recent relationship breakup or a job loss? Does it have anything to do with your gender identity or sexual orientation? Does it have to do with less obvious issues, such as your attempts to quit smoking or drinking? Are you feeling like a burden to your family? Are the issues more existential, such as doubting whether your life has meaning or whether you'll ever find joy?

Consider the costs and benefits of disclosing about these underlying issues: Will their understanding help them be supportive of you in the ways you need most? Or do you fear that the disclosures will be used against you, to force you into a hospital? These fears are not irrational, although in my experience people exaggerate the consequences of disclosing their suicidal impulses.

STRATEGY 3: Instruct your family members on how to respond

No one is born knowing how to help someone who is suicidal. It's particularly hard for parents, who may feel like they've failed. They may be under the mistaken assumption that talking with you about suicide will increase the chances that you'll do it, when in all likelihood the opposite is true.

You may have doubts about whether your parents, partner, or siblings can understand the triggers for suicidality from your viewpoint. Nonetheless, they may be more capable than you think. It may help for your relative to listen to and validate your feelings without offering advice, but you may need to be explicit about this. Consider this interchange between 25-year-old Randall and his mother, with whom he lived. She had found some of his diaries in which he had written fantasies about what would happen if he died.

RANDALL: I really would like to explain why I think about killing myself, but I don't think you'd want to hear about it.

MOTHER: Oh, come on, Randy. You know how much I care about you. I can't help if I don't know what's going on.

RANDALL: I'll tell you, but I want you to hear me out. I've been thinking about it almost daily, ever since I broke up with Josh.

MOTHER: (*Impatient*) Really? I thought you were over that! It was almost 6 months ago! You need to move on.

RANDALL: Mom, I know you feel that way, but you have to understand what is and isn't helpful to me at these times. It doesn't help to tell me to just move on. I need you to listen.

MOTHER: I am listening. But what can I do about it?

RANDALL: You don't need to do anything. Just listen. Ask me questions if you want to. I'd rather not get advice, however well-meaning.

MOTHER: Have you spoken with Dr. Ellis about this?

RANDALL: Yes, of course I have, and I'll continue to. But right now I want to talk to you.

MOTHER: (*Pauses*) OK, sorry. Tell me more.

RANDALL: That's good, that's what I need, more statements like that. I'm just really hurting, wondering if I should contact Josh again or if it's really over.

MOTHER: (*Frowns*) Don't do that . . . (*stops herself*). OK (*nods*), I get that. But what else? Why does this make you want to die?

RANDALL: Good question . . . (*pauses*). I just don't know how to keep going.

MOTHER: What do you want me to do when you feel that way?

RANDALL: Like I said, you don't need to do anything. Just listening and being there when I feel like talking is enough.

Notice that Randall has given his mother some instructions on what he needs, along with what he doesn't need. He reinforces her when she attempts to be a good listener. If she is able to stay with listening, he will begin to feel more trust for her.

STRATEGY 4: Discuss inpatient care

As described in the box on inpatient care (page 81), you and your relatives may feel differently about the need for hospitalization. If they think they can't ensure your safety, and no one else can either, then hospitalization is the best option, even if short term. Alternatively, it may be you who sees the need for inpatient care. In that case, educate your parents or spouse on what to expect (see the box on page 81). They will benefit from knowing that you're willing to go to the hospital (and which hospital your doctor or therapist recommends) and what will occur once you're there. Having this discussion when you are not in crisis works much better than trying to work it out in the moment when you're feeling desperate.

STRATEGY 5: Educate your relatives about what can feel demeaning or triggering

Usually, people with suicidal thinking do not respond well to bromides like "It will all get better soon" or "We only have one life to live." If you are not yourself religious, hearing religious views on suicide probably won't help either. You probably don't want to hear "You shouldn't feel that way," or "Look at all the people you're hurting." You may also be annoyed when relatives go into "doctor mode" and ask questions like "Do you have a plan? Or the means?"

These points may seem obvious to you, but remember that your relatives are feeling their way in the dark. If you find it awkward to educate them in this way, refer them to online resources for relatives and friends. An informative fact sheet is available at *www.rethink.org/advice-and-information/carers-hub/suicidal-thoughts-how-to-support-someone*.

Taking Stock

This chapter has emphasized specific strategies that you can incorporate into a suicide prevention plan. It helps to keep an updated version of this plan in printed form where you (and, if relevant, your relatives) can find it. If self-harm and suicidal thoughts are frequent, ask yourself what is and isn't working about the plan or what your relatives have done that has or hasn't helped.

Suicidality, however, can't always be addressed by distraction, support, or other behavioral strategies. It also concerns meaning and attachment and the way you think about your life and the world. When you feel like dying, everything can seem dark and bad, with the good or pleasurable parts of life receding into the background. Books from people who have lived through suicidal periods may be of considerable help, keeping in mind that everyone's journey is different. I'd recommend *Night Falls Fast: Understanding Suicide*, by Kay Jamison (2000), *Darkness Visible: A Memoir of Madness* by William Styron (1992), and *The Noonday Demon: An Atlas of Depression* by Andrew Solomon (2002). These are just a sampling of the large body of literature on suicidality and self-harm, which, although hard for many people to understand, are very common features of the human experience.

PART TWO

domains of life

DAILY ROUTINES AND STRESS

BD can be treated from a pharmacological, a psychotherapeutic, and a "lifestyle" perspective. You've seen how medications, therapy, and stress management strategies apply to reducing symptoms. What kinds of strategies contribute to improving quality of life in other domains, such as sleep, nutrition, or physical health? Interpersonal issues like family relationships and romantic attachments? What strategies help you optimize work and school functioning even when you have symptoms?

You will see two themes recurring in these next chapters. One concerns the critical importance of keeping regular sleep/wake cycles, even when environmental factors conspire to change them. Regularity in your nutrition and exercise routines also contribute to your mood stability and general health. The second theme has to do with negotiating relationships, whether those are within your family; in the dating, romantic relationship, or long-term couple realms; or at school or within the working world. BD can affect the quality of these life domains, but equally important are the effects that these domains have on you.

Part Two finishes with issues related to substance and alcohol use, a key problem for many people with BD. Daily routines and familial or social relationships are certainly relevant here as well: People tend to use substances at certain times of the day or night, with certain people, and in certain predictable social circumstances.

Throughout this part, I encourage you to self-observe—to keep track of your habits, understand how they came about, and consider your options—whether that means changing your habits or accepting things as they are and making the best of them. Adopting lifestyle management strategies—many of which have been tested in years of research as adjuncts to medications in BD—will almost certainly improve your quality of life.

6

strategies for healthy sleep

We should be able to expect normal sleep as part of being human, but many people (including me) find falling or staying asleep to be just out of reach. The reasons vary from one person to the other: stress, events that change our circadian rhythms, genetic factors, use of alcohol or drugs, anxious expectations, or simply having a barking dog in our midst.

Sleeping soundly is an experience few people with BD have ever had. Only 38% of people with BD are considered "normal sleepers"; others get either too little sleep or too much. Sleep disturbance can be both a trigger for mood recurrences and a symptom of existing episodes. In either case, poor sleep affects daytime performance, such as not being able to concentrate on a work or school assignment or stay awake during meetings.

It's important not to blame yourself for sleep problems (calling yourself lazy) given that they're caused by complex biological and psychological factors. Fortunately, there are things you can do to improve your sleep "hygiene," as it's called; concrete suggestions follow.

"Why Should Sleeping Well Require So Much Effort?"

Sleep hygiene means maintaining personal habits that over time contribute to your overall health and quality of life. First, there is the **importance of sleep/wake regularity**—staying on a consistent sleep and wake schedule even if you're not tired and not varying it by more than an hour from weeknights to the weekend.

Having a stable sleep/wake schedule is correlated with greater mood stability and a lower likelihood of mood episodes.

Second, it's easy to fall into the habit of spending hours in bed just thinking, which often turns into unpleasant ruminating. **Sleep restriction**, or minimizing the time you spend in bed without sleeping, is an important objective. So, if you wake up, start thinking and then worrying, it's best to get up for a while and relax so that when you hit the pillow again, you'll be ready for sleep. Third, **avoid napping** during the day (and especially in the early evening) to make up for lost sleep. Extensive napping is one of the leading causes of not being able to sleep at night.

Sleep problems are worsened when you're in an illness phase. When depressed, you may spend 12–16 hours in bed, and when you're manic, you probably won't want to sleep at all. As you might guess, the goal when depressed is to restrict your time asleep, and during mania or hypomania, to elongate sleep to fill out the normal 7 or 8 hours. Easier said than done!

Sleep is Not a Performance Piece: Prevention Strategies for Getting the Right Amount of Sleep

Despite our efforts to be conscientious about sleep, it's important not to view it as a performance that needs to be perfected. It's not like mastering a difficult piece of music or a sport. Sleep problems are often caused by inherited physiology, not much different from eye color or ear size.

The following strategies have been recommended by sleep researchers. Pick those strategies that you believe will work best, and if the first few don't work, take a break from them and try different ones. Avoid going into the night feeling like they'd better work or else. As you might guess, this kind of performance pressure can undo even the most sincere attempts at good sleep.

STRATEGY 1: Get a clear picture of your sleep difficulties

Sleep disturbances take a number of different forms:

- Not being able to fall asleep (primary insomnia)
- Waking in the middle of the night and not being able to fall back to sleep (middle insomnia)
- Waking too early (early insomnia)
- Sleeping too much (hypersomnia)

Pinpointing the nature of your sleep difficulties can be aided by a sleep diary that you fill out each morning. The daily sleep diary on page 102 is one such example. The diary is available as a mobile app (*https://consensussleepdiary.com*), which generates weekly graphs of your ratings of total sleep time, bed and wake times, and number of awakenings. There are other sleep apps that you may want to check out as well (for example, *www.sleepfoundation.org/wp-content/uploads/2024/03/ SF-23-127_Sleep_Diary_Interactive_03-2024.pdf*). Regardless of which method you choose, keep the diary over 2–4 weeks to help pinpoint where your difficulties lie. Then you may be able to answer questions, such as:

1. How would I best define my sleep problems? Trouble falling asleep, waking too often? Waking up too early and not being able to go back to sleep? Sleeping too much?
2. Am I budgeting enough time for sleep? Getting 7–8 hours?
3. Is my sleep schedule (bed and wake times) consistent or full of fluctuations?
4. Do I have more problems sleeping on school/work days than on weekends?
5. Do I tend to "sleep binge" on weekends (sleeping 10 hours or more) to catch up?
6. Am I spending significant time lying in bed without being able to fall asleep?
7. How long does it take in the morning for me to feel awake and alert?

STRATEGY 2: Track the potential causes of your sleep disturbances

A sleep diary can help you not only define the nature of the problem (or problems) but also keep track of what issues contribute to them. Contributory factors usually fall into one of three categories:

1. Your preexisting vulnerabilities: These can include having a history of insomnia, physical conditions like sleep apnea (see below), persistent anxiety or worries, fears related to your living situation (the neighborhood, privacy, whether doors are adequately secured), work stress, working variable shifts, or having a lot of time-changing travel. BD in itself is a vulnerability factor as can be the medications you take for it (such as having taken stimulants at the wrong time). The COVID-19 pandemic and restrictions contributed to a widespread vulnerability to sleep disturbance.

2. What's happening right when you're trying to sleep: Ruminating about

CONSENSUS SLEEP DIARY

Today's date:	Monday	Tuesday	Wednesday	Thursday	Friday	Saturday	Sunday
1. What time did you get into bed?							
2. What time did you try to go to sleep?							
3. How long did it take you to fall asleep?							
4. How many times did you wake up?							
5. In total, how long did these awakenings last?							
6. What time was your final awakening?							
7. What time did you get out of bed for the day?							

something that happened that day, having a room with too much lighting or an uncomfortable mattress, or a noisy neighbor. Your sleep can be disrupted by thoughts, emotions, or behaviors (drinking alcohol, smoking too many cigarettes, eating a heavy meal).

3. You can use the back of your sleep diary to record immediate causes of poor sleep or use any of the mood- or thought-charting tools covered in earlier chapters. You might record:

- Whether your sleep problems co-occur with feeling manic, hypomanic, or depressed. If your mood is spiking or deteriorating at the same time that you develop problems falling or staying asleep, then it is probably part of the bipolar syndrome. If the problems are persistent regardless of your mood, other factors are at play.

- Any negative thoughts that contribute to poor sleep, like "If I can't sleep, I'll get manic"; or "I'll be exhausted tomorrow and won't be able to handle the day." Has sleep become a performance venue? Record these thoughts.

- Medications that may be contributing to sleep problems or sleeping medications that cause a hangover the next morning.

- Alcohol or drug use from the day or night before.

Practical Measures to Prevent Poor Sleep Hygiene

Once you've identified the nature of your sleep problems and the probable causes, you can implement a number of research-supported strategies to improve your sleep hygiene. Then you can tackle more specific sleep problems that tend to be common in people with BD.

STRATEGY 1: Regulate your sleeping environment

Your bedroom should be dark, cool, and quiet. Keep the temperature at 60–70°F (15.6–21.0°C), making sure you aren't too warm or too cold in bed. Try to sleep on a comfortable mattress, not on the floor or on a couch. Although it may be comforting to share your bed with a dog or a cat, is it contributing to your ability to stay asleep? Your room should be dark or, at most, dimly lit. If you're very sensitive to light, use a sleep mask, especially during the early morning hours.

STRATEGY 2: Reduce noise during sleep times

If noise (barking dogs, traffic) is keeping you awake, try a white noise machine, ear plugs, noise-cancellation headphones, or some light music. You may have to get assertive with one of your neighbors if they or their pets are keeping you awake.

STRATEGY 3: Create a relaxing bedtime routine

This ritual can include low-key activities like taking a warm bath, reading a book, or listening to calming music—all activities that signal your body that it's time to wind down. If you suspect one element of your routine is keeping you awake (like watching the news), try experimenting by comparing sleep on nights with and without this element.

STRATEGY 4: Use relaxation techniques before bedtime

Before going to bed, try progressive muscle relaxation (*www.law.berkeley.edu/files/ Progressive_Muscle_Relaxation.pdf*), deep breathing, or meditation (such as the 3-minute breathing exercise on page 70). These strategies can help calm your mind and prepare your body for sleep.

STRATEGY 5: Avoid full meals, lots of liquid, and intense exercise within 3 hours before bedtime

Exercise is best done in the morning (to help you wake up) or in the late afternoon, before dinner. Eliminate coffee or other caffeine-containing substances (aspirin pain relievers, Sudafed) within 6 hours of bedtime. Watch how much alcohol or tobacco you consume before bedtime. Red wine, for example, may help you fall asleep but may also wake you up in a few hours.

STRATEGY 6: Limit use of phone or tablet screens 1–2 hours before bedtime

The blue light projected from your phone or tablet can interfere with the production of melatonin, a hormone that regulates sleep. Also, sending text messages or answering emails can increase your anxiety level, especially if they raise new problems that you'll have to address the next day. Make sure to turn off the notifications, buzzes, or blinking lights from your tablet or phone (such as by engaging the "Do Not Disturb" option on the iPhone).

Not all of these strategies will be practical for you, and avoid trying to implement them all at once. Try, for example, using a sleep mask and a white-noise generator for 2 nights. Then try 2 nights without screen use in the hours before bed and without your cat or dog on the bed. For each modification, determine the effects on your sleep patterns (how long it takes to fall asleep or how frequently you woke up) based on the consensus sleep diary (page 102). Eventually, you will be able to adopt those elements of the plan that work for you.

Getting Around Specific Sleep/Wake Obstacles Associated with BD

 TROUBLESHOOTING: "I always aim to go to bed early but stay up too late. Then I'm late to work and stressed out the next day. How do I change this pattern?"

Some people are "morning larks" (that is, they wake up early, refreshed and energetic, and usually go to bed early). Many people with BD are "night owls" with an "evening chronotype," which means that your circadian rhythms are primed to keep you up late. Your body secretes melatonin (the hormone that tells your brain that it's time to sleep) later in the evening, and your times of peak performance will be pushed into the afternoon. Being a night owl can be an advantage if your career requires late nights (musician or nurse), but it also goes along with sleeping later and, in some, experiencing "sleep inertia" in the morning (see below), which can interfere with work or school commitments. Unfortunately, owls are more prone to alcohol and tobacco use and to obesity. In the short term, having an evening chronotype also contributes to a chaotic sleep/wake schedule. Is there anything you can do to train yourself to go to bed earlier?

WORKAROUND 1: Figure out the chain of cause and effect

Let's apply a chain analysis to the problem of going to bed too late: Think about the sequence of vulnerabilities, immediate events, feelings, and thoughts that preceded going to bed. Imagine the following occurred:

10:00 A.M.: was late to work
10:00–6:00 P.M.: had stressful workday with conflicts with coworkers
6:00 P.M.: drank last cup of coffee
7:00 P.M.: went to gym
8:00 P.M.: got home and had a heavy dinner

9:00–11:00 P.M.: caught up on work assignments for next day
11:00 P.M.: had a phone argument with my partner
12:00 A.M.: watched a disturbing TV program
1:00 A.M.: checked my text messages
1:30 A.M.: went to bed (was targeting 11:30 P.M.)
2:00 A.M.: finally fell asleep
9:00 A.M.: woke up, already late for work

Any of these events could have contributed to going to bed later and having a poor night of sleep, but some probably had more effects than others. Which events in this chain could have been altered? You can change the timing of your last cup of coffee, when you exercised, or what you watched on TV. You can avoid using your computer or cell phone late at night, because bright lights (especially LEDs) can suppress your brain's production of melatonin and throw off your circadian rhythms, making it harder to sleep the next night.

Now examine whether any thoughts were associated with going to bed. Were you predicting that you wouldn't be able to sleep unless you went to bed later? Perhaps there was a thought like "Today sucked, and I worked really hard; I'll feel better if I give myself an hour or two of TV before I go to bed and face another day." That plan may have made you feel better in the short term but contributed to feeling exhausted and sleep deprived the next day. Try to examine these predictions and evaluate whether they proved useful, in the same way that you evaluated and challenged negative thinking in Chapter 1. Here are examples of the kinds of cognitions that tend to keep people awake:

"If I can't fall asleep right away, I'll be sunk the next day—I won't be able to concentrate and eventually I'll get fired."
"I'll have to drink coffee when I get home from work or else I won't get all that work done tonight."
"I won't be able to fall asleep unless I work out those issues with Anna [partner]."

Notice how many of these thoughts put performance pressure on you. You can overprepare for sleep in the same way that you can overprepare for an exam, a speech, or even a sexual encounter, and preparing can contribute to not being able to function. You can get into a vicious cycle in which you predict a poor night of sleep and then one occurs, which contributes to feeling poorly the next day, needing to nap, and then not being able to sleep the next night. You can start to "dread the bed."

Challenging these thoughts and, ideally, replacing them with alternatives will create a new chain that may lead to a different bedtime and wake time. For example:

"I don't need to get all of those assignments done tonight."
"I've dealt with poor nights of sleep before, and they don't necessarily ruin my next workday."
"Anna and I have some stuff to work out, but right before bed may not be the best time."

Modifying just a few links in the chain of events may lead to very different results.

⚙️ TROUBLESHOOTING: "I can't wake up in the morning. What can I do to wake up?"

Among the most difficult problems for people with BD is "sleep inertia," which refers to having reduced attention, memory, and energy for an hour or more after they awaken. Many people feel like there is a 100-pound weight on them when they wake up. They say, "I really try to get up, but I physically can't." I have heard this statement many times, and research shows that as many as 42% of people with BD report severe sleep inertia. Its main features are grogginess, impaired memory and attention, and a strong desire to go back to sleep, usually lasting about an hour. In BD it can be due to the cycling of moods, with more sleep inertia during depression and less during hypomania or mania. It can also be a warning sign of a new mood episode.

If you experience sleep inertia frequently, it's important not to come down too hard on yourself—sleep inertia is your body's way of saying you haven't slept well. There will be days when you will need to cancel work or school due to sleep inertia. If it can be arranged, a helpful accommodation is a later start to your workday.

WORKAROUND 1: Activate yourself upon awakening

People with BD who follow a program called RISE-UP for sleep inertia, in which they learn to activate themselves in the first waking hour, show significant improvements in the duration and severity of sleep inertia.

Start by giving yourself a full hour to awaken. During that hour, try the following:

1. Set your alarm clock away from your bed so that you can't turn it off without getting up. If you are prone to hitting the snooze button, set up two alarm

clocks at different places in the room. If you want a more effective (but annoying) alternative, look for a "Clocky" rolling or flying alarm clock that you have to chase around the room to turn off.

2. Dua Lipa? Lizzo? Program your phone to play some upbeat music when you awaken. If you don't like my choices, create your own playlist of songs or pieces that brighten your mood and play them while brushing your teeth, getting dressed, or making breakfast.

3. Do something physical within 1 hour of waking up: Walk the dog or stretch outside. Err on the side of physical instead of sedentary (such as reading the news) activities.

4. The hardest one: Jump in the shower and turn the water on cold or cool. You won't look forward to it, but it will definitely wake you up! A more modest alternative is just to wash your face, neck, and shoulders with cold water.

5. Expose yourself to sunlight. Weather permitting, have breakfast outdoors; if not, turn on the inside lights and open the curtains. If you can, do your exercises outside.

6. Have a conversation with another person, either face to face with a house-mate, or a phone or Zoom call to a friend or loved one.

You won't be able to do all of these on your first attempt, so mark the morning as a win if you've been able to do even one of them. Then try doing two of them for a week and increase to four if you can. Make sure to reward yourself for getting up and out earlier by going to your favorite store or coffee shop or doing an enjoyable activity after work or school.

WORKAROUND 2: Delay going back to bed

If the RISE-UP strategies are too difficult at first, set smaller goals and then work up. For example, when the alarm rings, get out of bed for 5 minutes before going back to bed. The next day, stay up for 10 minutes, and then 15 on the next. If you can, walk back and forth across your room for 5 minutes and turn on upbeat music. Having the coffee maker timed to start when your alarm rings will arouse your senses and make getting up a little more pleasant. At minimum, sit on the couch and read for 20 minutes to delay going back to bed.

WORKAROUND 3: Examine your self-talk

If you've been struggling with sleep inertia for a while, you may be unaware of the automatic thoughts coursing through your mind, such as "I should be able to hit the ground running" or "If I can't get up before 7, it means I'm lazy." Who says? The sleep disorders associated with BD can make it much harder to get up at a specific time, and people without mood disorders are not a fair comparison group. Self-accusations are not motivating. Try replacing them with self-talk that begins with "It's understandable that . . . I have trouble waking up, I'm fuzzy-headed in the morning, I have trouble getting to work on time." Add to the end of the sentence, "but I'm working on it." Once again, give yourself credit for intermediate goals, no matter how small.

WORKAROUND 4: *Involve others in the morning*

Many people dread the idea of interacting with someone first thing in the morning, even if it's their spouse or partner. Nonetheless, if you have a spouse/partner or a housemate with whom you share personal problems, ask them to conduct an experiment with you for 1 week, in which they agree to bring you a cup of coffee or tea in the first 20 minutes of the morning and sit with you and converse while you drink it. Figure out how you can reward the person later with a favorite meal, a movie, or another shared activity. After a few days you may be surprised to find that you wake up before the alarm rings and want to make the coffee yourself.

WORKAROUND 5: *Evaluate your medications*

A conversation with your physician may lead to some unexpected solutions. The first is determining whether your antidepressant, mood-stabilizing, antipsychotic, or sleep medications are contributing to sleep inertia. Some medications— particularly antipsychotics—can have a hangover effect, which is experienced as a lack of energy or mental acuity in the morning. Adjusting dosages, changing the timing of the medications to earlier, or changing to a different medication may help.

If you have attention-deficit/hyperactivity disorder (ADHD), you are most likely taking a stimulant in the morning that wears off by mid-afternoon. You can set your alarm for an hour before the time you want to be up, take your stimulant, and go back to bed. Then the stimulant will have kicked in by the time you want to wake. There is also a formulation of Ritalin called Jornay PM (methylphenidate hydrochloride) extended release, which you take in the evening so that its effects are felt in the morning. Stimulants have side effects—appetite suppression, increased heart rate and blood pressure, and irritability—and must be taken with an SGA or mood stabilizer. Discuss the pros and cons of each of these options with your doctor.

 TROUBLESHOOTING: "I wake up multiple times at night and can't get back to sleep. How do I change this pattern?"

There are many different reasons for "middle insomnia," or waking up throughout the night. It's particularly frustrating to have gone to some lengths to fall asleep, only to have it interrupted multiple times. The strategies you choose can vary depending on whether the cause is stress, a physical condition, eating or drinking habits, or other factors.

WORKAROUND 1: Rule out medical causes

Among the many possible causes of middle insomnia are sleep apnea and gastro-esophageal reflux disease. Sleep apnea is the intermittent closing and opening of the throat while breathing, often due to muscles in the back of your throat relaxing and blocking the flow of air into the lungs. Although it is often assumed to be an illness of older adults and the obese, it can also occur in young and healthy people and is common in people with BD. The symptoms include loud snoring, gasping for air, waking up with a dry mouth, headaches, irritability, and daytime fatigue. If your partner says you're snoring loudly (and especially if they say you sound like you're choking), talk to your doctor about getting a sleep study. This usually involves spending the night with electrodes on your scalp, chin, and chest that determine rapid eye movement (REM) and non-REM sleep, as well as breathing rate, air flow, blood oxygen, and heart rate (fortunately, you can do the overnight assessment at home). If you have sleep apnea, your doctor will probably recommend a continuous positive airway pressure (CPAP) machine, which blows air into your upper airway through a hose and face mask that you wear to bed.

Gastroesophageal reflux disease is characterized by heartburn, problems with swallowing, coughing, chest pain, and the feeling that you're regurgitating food. All of these problems are worsened when you lie down, contributing to middle insomnia. There are some simple lifestyle modifications that can help, including elongating the time between dinner and bedtime (aim for at least 3 hours), elevating your head on an extra pillow, and avoiding certain foods that trigger the reflux response. If these symptoms sound familiar, take the time to get a proper diagnosis from an ENT (ears, nose, and throat) specialist and discuss the treatment options with your doctor.

WORKAROUND 2: Avoid alcohol and substances

If you've been drinking a lot of wine or smoking cigarettes or cannabis before bed, there is a good chance it's contributing to intermittent waking. It may seem like a good idea to smoke weed in the middle of the night to sleep, but in all likelihood it will contribute to feeling dazed and groggy when you wake up.

WORKAROUND 3: *Monitor use of liquids and food before bed*

If you're waking up needing to urinate frequently, the cause may be lithium, which has thirst as a side effect. If this is the case, talk to your doctor about modifying the dose or changing the timing of the dose. Antipsychotics can cause constipation and some people need laxatives. If you're taking a liquid laxative (like MiraLAX) before you go to sleep, you have probably consumed at least 12 ounces of fluid, which will "come to call" in the night. There are other options for constipation that don't require drinking fluids (Ducolax or Senokot gummies or Metamucil wafers).

It's tempting to snack in the middle of the night, thinking it will help you sleep, but it probably won't. Also, you may be inadvertently training yourself to wake up in anticipation of food.

WORKAROUND 4: *Get up after 20 minutes*

The mantra "the bed is for sleeping and sex" is a good one to keep in mind; if you're spending more than 20 minutes in bed thinking or ruminating about daytime problems, then being in bed gets paired in your mind with worry. So, if you lie in bed for 20 minutes without falling asleep, get up for a while. Do some low-key relaxation exercises or meditation or take a quick shower. The ice water method (covered in Chapter 5) in which you dip your face in cold water for a few minutes can redirect your mind from worries to physical sensations.

WORKAROUND 5: *Consider sleeping medications*

Your doctor may recommend antipsychotics such as quetiapine (Seroquel) on an as-needed basis. Although they can certainly help you fall asleep, they have their disadvantages, including a worsening of morning sedation. Drugs like zolpidem (Ambien), lemborexant (Dayvigo), suvorexant (Belsomra), or Klonopin (a benzodiazepine) are other alternatives, but they are not meant to be taken over the long term because of their addictive potential. Also, people have been known to do unpredictable things in the middle of the night on these drugs, such as eat lots of candy or drive in their car without fully waking up.

 TROUBLESHOOTING: "Why do I feel like I need to nap several times a day?"

If you're not sleeping well at night, you may be playing catch-up during the day. It's certainly understandable to want to nap if you slept poorly, and a short nap midday can even help you overcome daytime drowsiness. But you can get into a vicious cycle where you nap frequently to catch up, such that daytime napping interferes with your sleep that night. Late-day or early evening naps especially decrease desire for nighttime sleep.

WORKAROUND 1: Determine your pattern of napping

Keep track of when and for how long you're napping throughout the week. Is it more than once a day? Is it consistently related to food—just after breakfast or after dinner? How is it related to the prior night's sleep?

WORKAROUND 2: Limit the scope and length of your naps

It may help to take a short nap at a break during your work or school day—this could even help you avoid sleep inertia the next day. But limit the length of the nap to 30–60 minutes and choose the same time every day so that it becomes part of your sleep/wake routine.

WORKAROUND 3: Choose an alternate activity to lessen fatigue

First, work toward reducing the amount of time you spend napping and then try to substitute another activity to fight fatigue. Light exercise, such as a walk in the neighborhood, can take the place of a nap, and when you return to your bedroom you may have less desire to sleep. Alternatively, close the door to your bedroom and spend half an hour eating outside, taking a shower, or doing some stretches.

How Family Members Can Help

If you are a young adult living with your parents, avoid getting them involved in your sleep/wake habits. Many young people have ongoing conflicts with well-meaning parents who constantly remind them to get to bed on time, or appear at their bedside with a gong the next morning. Managing your own sleep patterns is a great way to show your parents that you're capable of self-care without their intervention.

Your spouse or partner, however, can be of considerable help with sleep habits. If you share a bed, they can tell you whether you're snoring loudly (and whether you should get evaluated for sleep apnea). Your sleep habits may be "entrained" to theirs, such that you don't go to bed until they do or the reverse. If you and your spouse are having difficulty getting to bed on time, have a discussion with them about modifying the evening's routines so that bedtime comes earlier. This may require adjustments to dinnertime, TV time, whether or when you drink alcohol in the evening, or coordinating other nighttime activities.

If your spouse or partner keeps you awake because they have a different work schedule, or because they have meetings or social obligations at night, discuss with them some reasonable compromises: Can they schedule their Zoom or phone calls earlier, or in a room that's farther away from the bedroom, or use headphones to block out the sound of the respondent? If people are coming over late, can some of these social obligations be moved earlier or to the weekend? Explain that you're working on having more regular daily and nightly routines to manage your mood, which will probably be good news to them.

On the positive side, if your spouse is in bed before you, use their habits to modify your own. It may feel irritating to have to go to bed when they want to, but it may strengthen your relationship in the longer term to have similar sleep/wake routines.

Taking Stock

The form on page 114 will help you summarize the various causes of your sleep problems and organize the different remediation strategies. Go back through your sleep diary and determine which strategies worked the best for sleeping continuously and keeping a regular sleep/wake schedule.

If you're still having trouble with sleeping or waking, it's possible that you haven't identified all the links in the chain. Often missed are the thoughts that accompany sleep disturbance, dietary changes, and events that occurred yesterday or the day before that may be having a delayed effect.

Importantly, don't give up on yourself! Set realistic and achievable goals, rather than trying to change everything at once. Sleep habits develop over many years, and they take some time to change. On the brighter side, you may be surprised at the improvement in your mood when your sleep is deep, consistent, and uninterrupted.

SLEEP HYGIENE PLAN

The nature of my sleep disturbance (examples: being unable to fall asleep, waking too early):

Vulnerability factors (persistent anxiety, stressful job, travel across time zones, having variable work shifts):

Immediate factors (too much light in the room, uncomfortable bed, noise, partner who snores, dog that wakes me up):

Consequences the next day (sleep inertia, reduced effectiveness or concentration):

Chosen sleep strategies:

Strategies for dealing with sleep inertia:

7

effective communication with family members

Family relationships can strongly affect your ability to manage BD, both positively and negatively. When you're manic, family members can help you get the appropriate treatments, even though you may not want them at the time. When you're depressed, they can help you get back on your feet and believe in yourself again. They can remind you who you are when your self-esteem is at its lowest. Nonetheless, BD has special characteristics that make family conflict particularly intense. Family members know how to push our buttons.

Most of the time, family members are well-intentioned and just want to help, but in those attempts they may push you too far, becoming punitive when frustrated. They may express dissatisfaction with your progress or functioning or say (or imply) that you're too unstable to be trusted. All of this can make you feel like a child or, worse, a sick person who can't take care of themselves. For example, you may have a parent who is working excessively hard to get you to acknowledge the illness, comply with your medications and therapy, or adopt certain eating, sleeping, or exercise habits. As one patient of mine related, his mother "cornered" him before every therapy session with "Remember, we're paying a lot of money for this therapy. Go and bare your soul! Don't hold anything back."

Siblings can get into the mix, even if they're not physically present. If you're a young adult and still connected with your family of origin, you may suspect that your illness has elevated the status of your siblings within the family. They can come to represent the life you could have led if only you hadn't inherited a particular set of genes. You may feel like your family is ganging up on you.

I am defining family here loosely, to mean parents, a partner/spouse, siblings, or grandparents—generally, those with whom you live or are in close contact, even if your bed is elsewhere. Certain conflicts have a different meaning when with a parent compared to a spouse/partner, and I've flagged these examples accordingly.

The Power of Family Relationships

Since the early 1980s, I've studied families in which one person has BD, and the treatment I developed with my colleagues at UCLA, family-focused therapy (FFT), came out of this intensive study. We've found that people with BD are vulnerable to high levels of "expressed emotion" from parents or other relatives: high levels of criticism, hostility, or overprotectiveness. Living in a highly critical or hostile environment is not good for anyone, but it can put you at an increased risk for recurrences. On the positive side, people who receive mood-stabilizing medications and attend a course of FFT in which they and their family members share information about BD, develop relapse prevention plans and learn effective communication and problem-solving tools—including those described in this chapter—and have lower rates of illness recurrence and better life functioning over time.

Having family supports is just as important as taking medications for living well with BD. But to have appropriate supports, you have to work with your family members to share information about BD and resolve conflicts. That doesn't mean just bending to their will. It means coming to a common understanding of what to expect during your mood episodes, how they should respond to your symptoms, what they can do that is helpful, and in turn, how you can make life easier for them. In this chapter you'll learn some well-honed strategies for making things go better. The overall plan has three components:

1. Try to recognize when your buttons are being pushed.
2. Try to empathize with the emotional state of your family members and consider where their emotions are coming from. Recognize when their arguments or critical comments toward you, while hurtful, come out of their anxiety about your health or your (and their) future.
3. Develop a set of skills that will reduce conflicts and give you agency in determining your fate.

When facing family or couple conflicts that have occurred repeatedly, keep in mind the mantra "How can I do less of the same and more of something different?"

Preventing Conflicts from Escalating

 "I can't seem to control myself when my mom/dad/spouse/sibling irritates me—which is every single day. I'm always fighting with them. When they start criticizing me, I lash out."

Most people lash out at family members more regularly than coworkers, friends, or teachers, with whom there may be immediate negative consequences. Generally, family members won't fire or ghost us. However, you're paying a longer-term price for being continually angry at those with whom you live. How can you assert your independence and also have more constructive communication?

It's critical to recognize your family members' motivations, even if what they're saying and doing makes you feel crazier. In all likelihood they aren't trying to control you; they're afraid you'll have another episode, need to be hospitalized, die in an illness-related accident, or kill yourself. When they go on the offensive, it's best to show your understanding of these worries. The communication strategies listed below—while difficult to implement when you are in an illness episode or just plain angry—involve summarizing what your relative is worried about before giving your counterresponse.

STRATEGY 1: Use active listening

Imagine you're engaged in an angry back-and-forth with one of your parents concerning some aspect of your moods or behavior. You may feel quite irritated, but instead of thinking about your next salvo, try *active listening with paraphrasing*. Look at them, summarize what they've just said in your own words, ask questions to clarify their point of view, and nod your head occasionally. If you are in the height of mania or the depths of depression, you probably won't be able to respond in this measured way, but in between the extremes, active listening can give you considerable control over the direction an argument takes. It can also make your relative much more open to hearing your viewpoint.

For example, imagine your mom has gone after you about cursing too often, and your usual go-to is to say, "Fuck you." Instead, take a deep breath and try paraphrasing her ("You feel really hurt when I curse like that") or ask a clarifying question ("Are you saying that I always do that, or only when I'm in one of my moods?" or simply "How does it affect you when I do that?"). Be aware of whether you're letting her finish. You may be surprised at how this response slows things down and makes her think about her next comment. Then the stage is set for you to clarify your point of view without interruption. The table at the bottom of this page contains a number of paraphrasing statements that will help defuse conflicts.

 ## TROUBLESHOOTING: "What if I feel like I'm being attacked?"

It's especially hard to paraphrase a family member's statement if it feels like an attack. But consider how you can use active listening to shape the direction of a heated discussion. Robin, age 23, expressed a desire to discontinue her medications, and her father immediately reacted.

WORKAROUND: *Use active listening to turn the argument in a positive, collaborative direction*

DAD: Oh no, not this again! Why can't you just stick with your medications like your doctor says?

ROBIN: You're worried that I'm not taking them regularly.

DAD: Yeah, you know I am, and with good reason. Why aren't you taking them?

ROBIN: First, I am taking them. I haven't missed a dose in weeks. What I've expressed to you is that I feel ambivalent about them. You don't have to agree, but try to understand my reasons.

Using Active Listening in Conflictual Interactions

What they say	How you can paraphrase
"Did you take your medications today?"	"You're worried about me getting sick again."
"Do you think you should stay out so late?"	"You're concerned that lack of sleep will make me get manic."
"Don't you think you're jumping into this relationship too quickly?"	"You're worried that this relationship will hurt me somehow."
"I don't know what to say to you—nothing I say makes you feel better!"	"You're frustrated because you feel like you can't help me."
"You have to just buck up and beat this thing."	"You wish this was more under my control and that I could make it go away."

DAD: I've tried, and it doesn't make sense to me. You want to graduate college and get a job. Why would you play roulette with your future like that?

ROBIN: I understand your concern, and I share it to some degree. But I am discussing alternatives with Dr. _____ because the side effects have been very difficult for me. I need to make some long-term decisions about what dosages to take so that I can function at my usual level.

DAD: (*Softens*) I'm just worried because, well, you know, the last time you stopped them it was a disaster.

ROBIN: Yes, it was, and I don't want that to happen again either. But I'm looking for a compromise, not to do the same thing again.

DAD: I get that.

In this example, Robin has clarified why she feels mixed about her medications, which in this case were dosed too high. She was right to have questions about her regimen, and her father needed to understand the nature of her dilemma. Equally, he wanted to hear that she appreciated his concern. In this case, active listening fostered a sense of collaboration and reduced the potential for a fight.

STRATEGY 2: Make a positive request

If you want someone else to change their behavior, it's much easier for them to hear what you *do* want them to do than what you don't. When you're in conflict with a family member and it's your turn to talk, be clear but collaborative in getting across what you want: Look at the person (your spouse, parent, brother/sister) and say exactly what you want them to do and how it would make you feel if they behaved this way. The function of a positive request is to transition from criticism to problem solving. It allows you to express more positive emotions: those emotions you would feel if the problem were resolved.

Let's return to the example in which a parent expresses annoyance at your cursing. Imagine that you feel depressed, and your cursing reflects frustration that no one seems to understand your distress. You could say, "OK, I will do my best not to curse around you, but I'd appreciate it if you'd give me more room to express myself when I'm depressed—sometimes I just need to let off steam."

Consider the argumentative comments that you might be tempted to make when angry and how you can express the same content in a positive request form (see the examples in the table on page 120). You can also coach your family members to use positive requests with you. For example, if they react strongly to something you've said, coach them on how to let you know that they were hurt: "If I say

Examples of Positive Requests for Change

Critical or argumentative comment	Positive request for change
To your spouse: "I don't like your tone of voice."	"I'd appreciate it if you would use a kinder tone of voice with me."
To your spouse: "Your office is a sloppy mess."	"I'd feel relieved if you'd take responsibility for cleaning your home office each week."
To your parent: "I hate it when you remind me of my psychiatry appointments over and over."	"I'd feel more confident if you'd remind me of my appointments only once and then leave the rest up to me."
To your spouse: "You never cook dinner; you always leave it up to me."	"We should develop a plan for who cooks dinner on what nights so that it feels like a fair division of labor."
To your sibling: "Stop asking me about my moods the minute you see me."	"I'd appreciate it if when we see each other we talk about things other than my moods (give examples of other topics)."

something insulting, please alert me so that I can think of more productive ways to say it. I hope I can do the same with you."

 "Whenever I get that 'bee-like' face from my wife, I feel infuriated. She doesn't even need to say anything. I know what she's saying with it."

Not all communication is verbal. Sometimes we cut each other off or express our anger through nonverbal behavior. We often react strongly to well-known facial expressions or tones of voice in people with whom we're close. A simple movement of the mouth or rolling of the eyes can be misread as an attack. Individuals with BD, who have often been the target of critical comments from parents or other relatives, may be especially prone to misreading facial expressions, such as knowing when an expression reflects fear or anger. Certain nonverbal expressions ("eye rolling," for example), although usually seen as negative, may reflect the person's internal struggle over how to manage their emotions. Your relative may deny having made a face and accuse you of being overreactive. How do you avoid getting triggered in such situations?

STRATEGY: Check your pulse

When in conflict with a family member, it's usually best not to assume that you know what the other person is feeling. First, take a breath and delay your response by a few seconds. Ask yourself what you're feeling and whether you might be "projecting" your emotions (especially your anger or resentment) onto the other person.

Consider whether there might be other interpretations of their facial expressions. If you aren't sure, ask them what their look means, in as nondefensive a tone as you can muster ("Tell me what it means when you roll your eyes like that," or "I can see your facial expression just changed. What is it saying?"). Then you may be in a better position to talk through the problem.

 TROUBLESHOOTING: "What if they won't talk to me?"

If you've had a series of significant conflicts with your spouse, partner, or parent (for example, during or after a manic episode), they may have shut down so that you can no longer use your communication skills to break the impasse. There is no easy answer to this problem, and some relationships (including marriages) can go years with people avoiding each other. Sometimes this disconnection reflects a discrete negative event (for example, an infidelity) and at other times a series of less significant conflicts that have added up over time.

Sometimes a simple apology can get people talking again. If your relationship with your parents, spouse, or other family members has recently gone quiet, consider one of the repair strategies discussed in Chapter 4. Here are some examples:

> "I think you're pretty angry with me. I'm sorry if I've hurt your feelings. I'd like to get us talking again."
> "I'm not used to us being so disconnected. That must mean I've hurt you. Can we talk about it?"

These strategies are difficult because they require putting your own anger aside. Also, they may not clear the air right away. Be patient—people often need time to absorb apologies. Also, once your relative starts talking again, you may get an earful. That's a point at which your active listening skills will come in especially handy.

 "I get infuriated by my siblings, especially when anything about my illness comes up."

In the early 1950s, before the advent of lithium, clinicians made observations about what people with BD reported about their childhood environments. Many reported that their siblings envied them because of their talent, intellect, high energy, or personality. Then, when the person with BD became ill, siblings relished their new role as the healthy, functional ones in the family.

Siblings can come to represent the life you could have had if you hadn't become ill. What they've achieved, in terms of their job, home life, or educational opportunities, can generate excessive praise from your parents and feel unfair to you. It can feel doubly unfair when siblings want to play a "parentified" role in your treatment. If you're facing these dynamics, you probably feel resentful of your siblings, and they may not have a clue as to why.

STRATEGY 1: Remind yourself of things you've been able to do that your sibs can't do

Are your siblings' lives really carefree? Haven't they had difficult times? There's no need to point this out to them, but be aware that they may feel competitive with you for long-standing reasons they can't explain. At a minimum, they may secretly resent that your parents expend so much effort on your health, wondering whether the same would have been done for them.

STRATEGY 2: Ask yourself if you are taking out your anger on them

Is your anger really at your sibling, or is it at your parents, who (advertently or inadvertently) pit you against each other? Try to distinguish what is being evoked in the here-and-now versus what are old sibling rivalry issues. At some point, perhaps when you're stable and things are going better between you and them, consider discussing these issues openly. Ask them whether they're aware of imbalances in your relationship. You may be surprised to find that they have their own envy, jealousy, or admiration of you, even if unexpressed.

 "I feel like my spouse/parents don't understand my illness. They don't trust me and want to control me. They say I'm too sick to make decisions for myself. Then I get angry, and they say 'See, you're not stable.'"

This situation is one of the most volatile for people with BD. You may be justifiably upset by something that just happened (for example, a sibling said something you found insulting). Perhaps you got angry and your parent followed up with "Have you talked to your doctor about getting a medication for that?" One patient of mine explained, "When I tell my folks about something that upset me at work, they immediately jump to 'Have you taken your lithium today?'" Responses like this can feel very dismissive, especially when you feel that your emotional reactions are valid and within the norm.

Here are some preventive strategies to consider. They have one element in common: sharing what is and isn't true about BD. These strategies are best implemented when you and your family members are calm, because they involve mutual collaboration.

STRATEGY 1: Educate them on the basics of BD

You are the expert on this illness, having gone through it and knowing what happens to you internally during manic and depressive episodes. If you haven't had extensive conversations with family members about mood symptoms, illness course, causes, and treatment, help get them informed. You can start with a handout for family members like the one on pages 124–126 or recommend readings, podcasts, or support groups (see, for example, *www.dbsalliance.org*).

STRATEGY 2: Educate them about how the bipolar label applies to you

Help them understand the difference between who you are (your personality, how you have always expressed yourself, the things that you care about) and your symptoms of depression or mania so that they don't label everything as a symptom. The table on page 127 contains examples of things my patients have said to their family members to explain their disorder when they feel they are being unfairly labeled. Notice the use of active listening and positive requests for change in these examples.

STRATEGY 3: Explain your position on medications

To be fair, sometimes a spouse or a parent repeatedly asks about medications because they rightly suspect that you haven't been taking them. If you've stopped one or more of your meds, be honest with them. Do they understand why you've gone off? Maybe you have good reasons, such as side effects or the drugs' ineffectiveness. If so, explain your reasoning to them. They will probably feel more at ease with your decision if they know you've discussed it with your psychiatrist and a plan is in place for "rescue medications" should you develop prodromal symptoms. Chapter 13 is devoted to the issues relevant to adopting a medication regimen.

STRATEGY 4: Consider family therapy

If these discussions with your family members or your spouse are coming up repeatedly and the fights are getting worse, consider getting some family or couple therapy from a provider who knows about BD. People often bristle at the idea of

An Informational Handout on Bipolar Disorder for Family Members

WHAT IS BIPOLAR DISORDER?

People with bipolar disorder (BD) have severe mood swings from states of excessive activity and energy (mania) to severe depression. The disorder affects about one in every 50 people, and usually starts in adolescence or young adulthood. It can continue throughout the life span but often gets easier to cope with over time.

WHAT ARE THE SYMPTOMS?

If I have bipolar I disorder, I can get depressed or fully manic. These are states of about 1 week to several months in which I become overly happy and excited or overly irritable and angry. I may feel like I can do things that no one else can do or that I'm a very important person. When I'm in this state I sleep less than usual or not at all, have an unusual amount of energy, talk fast and jump from one idea to another, do too many things at once, and get easily distracted. I may do things that are risky and impulsive, like spending a lot of money or driving recklessly. If I have bipolar II disorder, I won't have full manias but I'll have less intense periods of heightened activity and decreased sleep called hypomanias, alternating with periods of depression.

When I get depressed, the opposite occurs: I get low or very sad in mood, lose interest in most things and most people, have little motivation to do things I usually enjoy, have trouble sleeping (even though I desperately want to) or sleep too much, have little or no appetite, and get fatigued or low in energy. I may have ideas about ending my life or harming myself in some way. I may seem like I'm moving and thinking very slowly. These periods can last anywhere from 2 weeks to several months.

In the periods after a manic, hypomanic, or depressive episode, I need time to convalesce and get back to my ordinary self. During the periods in between I may function well but I may have to cope with minor symptoms of depression, mania, or anxiety and worry.

(continued)

HOW WILL BD AFFECT THE FAMILY?

When I become ill, I may have trouble relating well to people in the family. I may get irritable or angry easily in manic states, especially if people want to stop me from doing things I want to do. I may get irritable during depression, especially when people work too hard to get me to be active. At times I may be hard to motivate and won't respond when asked to do something. It's important at these times to use healthy family communication skills, such as active listening or making patient and diplomatic requests, acknowledging one another's viewpoints. If our family is having a lot of problems, we may benefit from some family counseling.

WHAT CAUSES BD, AND WILL ANYONE ELSE IN THE FAMILY GET IT?

BD runs in families, but if one person has it, the chances that another first-degree relative of that person (a son or daughter or a parent or sibling) will get it is about 10–15%. The symptoms are probably caused by dysregulations in circuits of the brain involved in emotion regulation. Episodes can also be triggered by stress, including family conflicts or life events, especially events that disrupt my sleep. No one chooses to become bipolar but there are many things that can be done to stabilize it.

HOW IS BD TREATED?

I need to see a psychiatrist for medications. They prescribe mood stabilizers (examples are lithium, valproate [Depakote], or lamotrigine [Lamictal]) or certain antipsychotic medications (for example, aripiprazole [Abilify], risperidone [Risperdal], quetiapine [Seroquel], lurasidone [Latuda], cariprazine (Vraylar), or lumateperone [Caplyta]). Taking an antipsychotic does not mean I am psychotic, because these medications are used for mood stabilization as well. My doctor may also recommend an antidepressant medication to improve my mood and sleep. I need to see my psychiatrist at least once a month to make sure I am getting the right dosages, to have my blood levels tested, and to get control over the side effects. These medications can be hard to take (for example, some of them cause hand tremors or weight gain), and I may go through periods of not wanting to take them.

(continued)

If my symptoms get severe or if I feel like I'm going to hurt myself, I may need to be in the hospital for a short time. Being in the hospital is nothing to be ashamed of; it can be very helpful in reestablishing periods of stability and getting my medications readjusted.

I should also see a therapist to help me develop skills for managing my mood swings and to cope with events that could contribute to recurrences. Many people learn to recognize early warning signs of new episodes and get help before their symptoms get out of hand. Our family may benefit from counseling to learn more about BD and how it affects me, and to learn to communicate effectively when I am having episodes. Sometimes, therapy comes in the form of groups with other individuals with BD, or with other families coping with it.

When I am depressed, some regular exercise may help lift my mood, either alone or with another person. However, I may not want to exercise when I am feeling low, so it's important to let me do it at my own pace.

WHAT DOES THE FUTURE HOLD?

There is every reason to be hopeful. With a regular program of medications, therapy, exercise, and family support, my episodes will become less frequent and less disruptive. I can still reach my personal goals and have a successful work and family life. Many very talented and creative people have had this disorder.

Constructive Responses to Educate Family Members

The situation with family members	Things you can tell them
You are in a depressive episode and are having trouble meeting their demands.	"I am in a state of depression right now. That means I have low energy, fatigue, and limited concentration. I'd appreciate it if you can reduce your expectations while I'm recovering."
Your relatives are making critical comments and implying that the illness is all under your control.	"I know that you feel that way, and right now I'm doing a lot of my own self-critiquing. Instead of telling me what you don't like, tell me what you want me to do differently."
They are asking you lots of questions about medications, therapy, or other aspects of your psychiatric care.	"I understand that you're quite concerned, but I have to make my own choices. I'm discussing these topics with my doctors. I want to be able to discuss other things with you."
They are continually calling your doctor to encourage them to raise your medication dosages.	"I understand that you've been in contact with Dr. _____ about my medications. I would really appreciate you telling me first before you call them so I can know what medical decisions are being discussed. It's important for me to be in control of my own treatment."

going to family or couple therapy, thinking that it will be a sophisticated way of blaming them for their family's problems. In fact, the most effective family and couple intervention strategies are psychoeducational, dealing directly with what BD is, how it affects members of the family, and how the reactions of your family members (or spouse/partner) affect you.

Chapter 14 contains more in-depth information about family or couple therapy. If you are able to find a suitable therapist, ask the clinician to help you clarify for your family members what the illness is and is not and what they can do to be helpful. If you can't find an appropriate provider, consider attending a Depression and Bipolar Support Alliance (DBSA) group (*www.dbsalliance.org*) together, or a National Alliance on Mental Illness family support group (*www.nami.org*).

In-the-Moment Strategies for Dealing with Family Conflict

 "When I get into it with my family, I lose it really quickly. What do I do right then?"

When your discussions with your relatives look like they're headed in the wrong direction and you've tried some of the strategies above, consider the following:

STRATEGY 1: Use the three-volley rule

When your partner, spouse, or parent has criticized you and you've responded, and then they criticize you in a different way (or amplify the first criticism) and you've responded to that, and then they come up with a third critical comment, it's time to walk away. Say (as gently as possible), "I'm done with this conversation for now. We can discuss it later on, when we're both more coolheaded." You can even cut it off after two volleys if it's going in a predictable direction. If they start following you around the house to keep the conversation going, stop, breathe, and say, "I think this conversation has run its course and it's not helping. I'm getting upset, so let's put this off until later." Then stop responding.

STRATEGY 2: Give yourself a time-out

As you know from earlier chapters, you can use awareness of your moment-to-moment internal state to guide your choices. If you're already irritable, this is not the time to have a showdown with your family. If you're in the midst of a negative exchange and feel like you're losing control of your emotions, or like you're going to hit someone or break something, give yourself a time-out. Tell your family members that you need some breathing room. Then exit the confrontation and go into another room to do a 3-minute breathing exercise (page 70), listen to music, punch a pillow, or otherwise distract yourself before your next interaction with them.

Imagine returning from work or school feeling agitated or anxious and your spouse or parent asks, "How was your day?" Perhaps you respond minimally (such as "It was OK") and they get intrusive: "Did you ask for the raise? Are they going to give you some time off?" When you feel the heat rising, it's a great time to excuse yourself to cool off. Promise to come back to discuss your day when you've had a moment to relax.

In this example, Dustin (age 35) has recently returned to his job after a 3-month interval of depression from which he hasn't fully recovered. When he gets home, his wife, Cassie, wants to check in with him.

CASSIE: How was work today, honey?

DUSTIN: The usual. (*Quiet, puts coat on rack*)

CASSIE: Did you have that talk with Antonio [boss] you were going to have?

DUSTIN: Yeah, sort of.

CASSIE: So how did it go?

DUSTIN: (*Pauses*) I'd rather not get into it.

CASSIE: Oh, no, that means things went badly. What happened?

DUSTIN: Like I said, I don't want to get into it. How about after dinner I can tell you all about it.

Notice that in this case Dustin doesn't blow off Cassie, nor does he indulge her with what she wants to know. He is hungry and already irritated and knows it won't go well. But it would also be important for Dustin to explain to her later what happened with his boss. If both Dustin and Cassie are familiar with active listening, he can tell the story while she listens, empathizes, and asks questions. Then it is her turn to disclose what she's worried about ("I'm worried that you'll get fired") while Dustin listens.

Taking Stock

The strategies outlined in this chapter depend on relationships that are at least civil. If your relationship with family members has become threatening or abusive, get some distance from the other person, even if it means living elsewhere for a time.

If you've been able to try out some of these strategies, evaluate what has and hasn't worked. What responses seem to calm you down without inflaming your family members further? How can you do less of the same and more of something different?

If you want to record your use of the strategies systematically, create a chart with columns like the following:

- In the last week, what situations with your family members made you angry? With which family members?
- What thoughts went through your mind?
- How did you express your anger?
- What were the consequences of this confrontation for you and them (such

as a broken glass, a slammed door, threats, a ruined cell phone)? Were anyone's feelings hurt?

- What alternatives do you have for the next time? How can you change the
  sequence of events that lead to these interchanges?
- Are there any other communication skills (for example, active listening)
  you could have used?

Importantly, keep trying. Good family and couple relationships are essential
to your emotional and physical health. Relationships don't change readily, but they
can be adapted when both sides make consistent efforts to collaborate. Be aware of
your mood states when entering into confrontations that typically have not gone
well. Saying, "I don't want to get into this right now, but we can talk later" is a per-
fectly reasonable response to head off conflicts.

8

thriving with a partner

DATING, SEX, AND LONG-TERM RELATIONSHIPS

BD can affect your romantic and sexual relationships in ways you may not be able to predict. In turn, stressful romantic relationships can affect the course of your mood symptoms. Recognizing how your illness contributes to or is influenced by close relationships can only help when you meet a new person or in keeping a long-term relationship going. BD does not have to be a "third person" in a couple.

Chapter 7 covered day-to-day communication strategies for defusing conflicts in families, focusing mainly on parents or siblings. Here the subject is your relationship with an intimate partner—from the encounters that start a new relationship to the problems that emerge in long-term partnerships. Living well in this domain of life means knowing the best way to explain the disorder to someone you've just met (often an anxiety-producing task), how to react to their attitudes about mental illness (which may include stigmatizing statements), and how to deal with your moment-to-moment shifts in mood when you're with them. If you're married or have a longtime partner, you can't prevent every argument or tense interaction, but there is a role for in-the-moment regulation of your moods so that you're less likely to overreact to relationship events. In turn, you can coach your partner on how to discuss problems in ways that are less stigmatizing and likely to elicit your mood swings.

Strategies for Avoiding Risky or Unwanted Sexual Encounters

 "I'm feeling like I want to have sex with everybody. How do I allow myself to be free and my life to be exciting without getting hurt by my impulses?"

If you're just starting to date after a long hiatus, you may be familiar with the desire to have a lot of sex with many different people. This desire is amplified during hypomania or mania and usually goes along with feeling extra confident and attractive and underestimating the risks and overestimating the rewards of sexual intimacy. Everyone has their own rules, beliefs, and personal boundaries about sex, but mania has a way of throwing them all by the wayside.

If you're just coming out of a depressive episode, you may overrespond to the novelty of a new partner, even if you barely know them. A study of people with BD who were dating online found that 65% reported regretting their risk-taking behavior related to online dates (such as sending photos privately), compared to 31% of people without BD.

PREVENTION STRATEGY: Protect yourself

Determine your mood state before you go out at night, either by consulting your mood chart or by taking stock of any recent symptoms (such as not needing as much sleep as usual). If you're in the mild/moderate hypomania or mania range, your inhibitions are down and you're more likely to have a spontaneous sexual encounter. Much like alcohol, being "under the influence" of mania or hypomania can make others seem more attractive, and a sexual encounter that you would ordinarily never consider can seem very enticing and devoid of risks. Here are some ways to protect yourself:

1. If you're going out to a club, party, or bar, take along someone you trust. Instruct that person to drive you home (or call a cab or Uber) if you're behaving impulsively (being overtly flirtatious or suggestive with strangers, for example). Ideally your trusted person will be a close friend, someone who understands your diagnosis.

2. As always, take along condoms. When dating, many people (bipolar or not) find themselves in unexpected sexual encounters in which their partner seems

unconcerned about pregnancy or sexually transmitted diseases. Your judgment is likely to be impaired when hypomanic or manic, so it's best to protect yourself and the other person.

3. Understand that, even if you're taking mood stabilizers, certain drugs (cannabis, ecstasy, alcohol, cocaine) will accelerate your sexual desire. Avoid accepting drinks from strangers unless you've seen the bartender pour it and hand it to you.

4. Avoid going out when sleep deprived. Certain aspects of dating may not mesh well with your attempts to manage your daily rhythms. Meeting new people may mean staying up much later than you intended, drinking more, sleeping at someone else's house, or any number of other changes in routines that, while temporarily rewarding, can contribute to mood instability and risky behavior. That doesn't mean you shouldn't date but be cognizant of what you can and can't tolerate.

IN-THE-MOMENT STRATEGY: Wait a few hours and see if you're still tempted

Sometimes just buying yourself time will help you avoid unwanted sexual encounters. If you're feeling elevated and someone is coming on strong, look at your watch or phone and see if you can wait a few hours. Ask yourself, "If it's nine o'clock, will I still want to be with this person at eleven?" If you internally respond with, "I can't wait that long—I need to go with this person now or they'll find someone else," that's a clue that you are doing something that is discordant with your longer-term desires.

Disclosing Your Diagnosis

 "No one will want to go out with me once they know about my disorder."

The interval following an acute episode, particularly if it required hospitalization, will make you acutely aware of others' judgments about psychiatric labels. You may become more attuned to the off-the-cuff statements that people who are not bipolar make routinely, such as "I'm really bipolar today," "I was 'manic cleaning' all weekend," or "Too bad I didn't take my lithium." You may fear that others will reject you as soon as they find out about your illness. Kay Jamison, in her wonderful autobiography *An Unquiet Mind*, warns readers to take medicines out of the medicine cabinet before having guests over for dinner or lovers spend the night, lest they find out that you're taking lithium.

Some people with BD think this is a nonissue, because someone who won't date you because of your illness is not worth knowing anyway. Although that's a reasonable position, it's hard to know what people do and don't understand about BD before the topic comes up. Maybe they've had a parent or former partner with the disorder, or associate BD with movies they've seen where the main character is bizarre and dangerous.

The stigma of various psychiatric disorders is very real. Many people have mistaken beliefs about the dangers of BD, such as "People with BD are violent," "You can't (or shouldn't) have children," or "You can't work or have a successful career." Others have a positively biased view, thinking that you must be extra creative or talented or that being with a person with BD will be an exciting rollercoaster ride. Of course, much of how your intended partner understands the disorder will be based on what you tell them and when.

PREVENTION STRATEGY: Decide on when and with whom to disclose your BD

There is no rule of thumb for disclosing your disorder in a new relationship. I've had many discussions with my patients on this issue, and they're evenly divided on telling new partners right away or waiting until the relationship feels like the real thing. If you have ongoing symptoms, disclosing your disorder to a potential partner may help explain mood swings or anxiety that you may experience in their presence. You may learn a lot about their attitudes on mental health: Do they spontaneously mention someone they know with a psychiatric illness? They may ask, appropriately, how they would know if you were cycling into an episode and what they could do to help. You may feel better being with a person who knows your secrets; it can build trust.

There are also disadvantages to immediate disclosure. It may be "too much information" for a first or second date. You may learn that they hold stigmatizing attitudes ("Am I safe with you?"). If confidentiality is important to you, you may not be certain that this person will keep it private. If you are unsure about these things, it may be best to wait until you know the person better.

If you're thinking about telling a new partner about your BD, try the decision tool in the box on the facing page. Whereas the responses are just an illustration, they may help you organize your thoughts about a person you are dating.

Decision Tool for Disclosing Your Diagnosis

Who I'm thinking of telling: *Kaitlin*

Why do I want her to know?

I just started dating her, and I'm still depressed. I want her to know why I don't always call her back or why I sometimes sound unenthusiastic.

What are the advantages of telling her now?

1. *She needs to understand my behavior if we keep going out.*

2. *She asked me why I seemed uninterested and withdrawn on Saturday.*

What are the disadvantages?

1. *What if she can't deal with it and ghosts me?*

2. *Maybe it's too soon to tell her something so personal; she hasn't told me that much about herself.*

How do I want to explain it?

I get depressed sometimes, really depressed, and when I'm like that I may sound like I'm not interested in what you have to say. It's not you—I really like you, and what you say is interesting to me. When I get like that, everything makes me tired, and I get slowed down. Other times I get super excited and over the top, and then everything seems interesting. I don't always feel this way—it comes and goes. That day I was in a bad patch.

IN-THE-MOMENT STRATEGY 1: There are some good ways to explain BD

Let's imagine you are in the early phases of a relationship, and you're feeling the need to reveal your health history. You're eager to find out if it will be a deal-breaker for the person you're getting to know. You may be having symptoms that you feel a need to explain, or perhaps they've asked you whether you see a therapist or take medications. They may have observed that you have trouble sleeping. Alternatively, they may have told you about their own mental health problems, and not telling them about your own may feel disingenuous. These are all good reasons to be up-front. What are some good ways to explain it?

One person with BD put it like this:

"I take the angle that is most grounded. I don't like to give a superficial explanation or be flippant about it, because then I'm adding to the stigma. I give enough detail so that they know what I'm talking about—not just the symptoms but also how I found out that I had it, what effect it's had on my life, and what I do to try to prevent episodes. I also want to have an understanding of where they're coming from, what their misunderstandings are."

The box on page 135 gives one example of how to explain it. Here is another way:

"I want you to know something about me so that my behavior makes sense to you. I have bipolar disorder, which means that sometimes I'll have moods that go from extreme highs to extreme lows. When I have high periods, I feel on top of the world and full of all sorts of plans. I don't need to sleep. I may get irritable and full of energy. When I'm depressed, I have trouble getting motivated to do ordinary things, or I sleep a lot and feel sapped of energy. I'm taking mood stabilizers, and I get regular therapy. Most of the time I'm OK, and I'm the person you see in front of you. But when I'm in these episodes I may do or say things that are hurtful, or I might be hard to connect with. Do you know much about bipolar disorder?"

This person avoids details about hospitalizations, delusions, or police contacts, which are not essential at first. They avoid using pejorative terms (*bizarre, crazy, whacked out*) and communicates an essential point: "I am not my disorder—it's something I have, but it's not the sum total of who I am."

IN-THE-MOMENT STRATEGY 2: What to do to manage their reactions

People you meet (and even your own relatives) don't necessarily know much about BD, and you may have to educate them (see the educational handout on pages 124–126). Partners may have immediate reactions like "Whoa! That's intense!" or "My ex-wife is bipolar," or "I wish you'd told me sooner" (Why?). You may feel them pulling away. If you sense this, it's important to avoid overreacting. Yes, there is stigma about the disorder, and it's unfair, but your new partner may need time to process what you've just told them. Their reactions are likely based on fear. Ask them whether they want to know more about it. Provide reassurances; if appropriate, communicate that you like and appreciate them, recognizing that they need to make their own choices.

If you disclose your disorder to a person who then ghosts you, it stands to reason that you don't want that person in your life. They will not be supportive if you have a new episode. They may lack empathy, and may run away from other life problems as well. If you want to meet other people with BD who have navigated the dating world, this might be a good site for you: *www.BipolarDatingSite.com.*

 "The person I'm dating seems to be all about my illness."

Your new person may react in the opposite way as well: They may want to rescue you. They may react to the disclosure of your BD with excessive empathy: "I totally understand and accept you, and appreciate you even more now; I feel terribly for you, I can only imagine how difficult this has been; I want to be there for you." From that point on they may check your emotional temperature frequently (asking how you're doing, if you're OK that day). If you've been expecting rejection from someone you've started dating, this kind of reaction may be a relief, but it may also raise red flags. Why is the person bending over backward to show their understanding?

There are people who feel empowered by being with someone who has emotional turmoil. They may be quite compassionate and caring people, but they may also be excited by the dramatic ups and downs of BD. Taking care of a partner with BD may give them a sense of control and guard against their own feelings of inadequacy. A healthy relationship, of course, is one where the two people are on equal footing.

If you sense these dynamics operating but you like the person otherwise, give it time. At some point you may want to point out: "I appreciate how compassionate you are, but I also want you to know that I don't need to be rescued. . . . I have doctors, family members, and friends who can help me . . . what I want in my personal life is an equal relationship."

 "My mood shifts over the course of a date."

Dating can take turns for the better or worse when your mood is unstable. Having an unstable mood doesn't mean you shouldn't date, but think preventively about how you can minimize the effects of your moods when going out with a new (or reasonably new) person. Check in with yourself before you go out for the evening: What are your moods telling you that you do or don't want to do? Get more seriously involved or keep a distance? Talk to your date about your disorder? Make the evening short because you're feeling fatigued? Do something that doesn't require long periods with heavy conversation?

PREVENTION STRATEGY 1: Give yourself an out

When you start dating someone, your excitement may build at first and then crash over the course of a single evening. This is not an unusual experience for people with BD. If you're out with someone and depression or anxiety reaches a certain level, you may feel like you can't wait for the evening to be over. This feeling may not be a reflection of how you feel about the person as much as it is mental exhaustion, which colors how everything looks. This is a good time to give yourself an out, which may require some planning.

One option is to tell the person you're not feeling well ("It must be something I ate"). If you prefer, tell the truth: you're feeling anxious and now is not a good time for you to be out; you'd like to make an early evening of it, and you want a raincheck. There is nothing wrong with this—you are empowering yourself by deciding what you can and can't tolerate. Of course, you may be far from home when this happens. If you are not going to drive yourself, work out a plan in advance to be picked up by a close friend or family member. At minimum, take along a credit card and a rideshare app (such as Lyft or Uber) to make sure you get home.

Later, once you've had a chance to reflect, consider what happened that evening that contributed to wanting to go home early. Perhaps the person said something that alluded to your disorder and made you feel inadequate. You may have exaggerated the negatives of a certain conversation (such as thinking you were coming across as dull or pessimistic). You might be telling yourself that having BD makes you a less attractive person than your date. Be aware that you're having those thoughts and question whether they are *useful*: Do they help you understand how you feel about this person? Do they help clarify what you do or don't want to do the next time you see them?

When pessimistic self-talk emerges, sit for a few minutes, breathe, and observe the thoughts from a decentered stance: "I'm having that thought at this moment, that I like (your date's name) but can't imagine being with them. I wonder what brought it on? What am I feeling in my body? What other thoughts or images are present?"

IN-THE-MOMENT STRATEGY: Think about how you are coming across

If you feel elevated or hypomanic during a date, it's easy to come across as too forward, excited, or carried away with thoughts of a new love. An ordinary person may seem like the one you've always been looking for. You may be tempted to say something very intimate or forward right away. It's best to err on the side of not doing or saying things that may seem extravagant or presumptuous.

If you have ascertained that you started the evening in an elevated or anxious state, do a self-assessment: Am I talking too loudly or too much? How was my sleep last night? Is this evening generating unrealistic fantasies about how life could be with a new person? Am I saying these things out loud? You can also do a reality check with your partner: "I'm feeling awkward. Am I talking too much?" "I'm sorry, did I cut you off?" "It's been a while since I've dated and I'm a bit rusty." You may be surprised to learn that they think *they're* talking too much.

Maintaining a Good Long-Term Relationship in the Fallout of an Episode

Longer-term relationships bring up a different set of issues for people with BD. Some of these issues bode well for new partnership—people with BD are capable of intense attachments and compassion for another person. The key relationship problem experienced by many with BD is how to express their emotional ups and downs with their partner, and in turn, how their partner responds to emotional volatility.

The interval following a mood episode is a particularly fraught time for couples. You may still be symptomatic but increasingly capable of self-care, and begin to feel overcontrolled by your partner, who is constantly asking you if you've taken your medications. Your partner may feel resentful that your episode has caused a disruption in both of your lives, or that you aren't taking better care of yourself. There may have been events during manic episodes that threaten the future of the relationship, such as impulse-driven infidelities or excessive spending. Once you have remitted, you may be able to talk openly about these events with your partner, with the recognition that it takes time to heal. The effects of depressive episodes on long-term relationships are less predictable. It can be harder to tell when a depressive episode has lifted; in the weeks after the worst of the episode, you may feel better but not yet able to engage in previously enjoyable activities with your partner. You may be less responsive to physical, sexual, or emotional attempts at intimacy. Your partner may become frustrated that you aren't more available, which can make you feel worse.

The principles we've already discussed in relation to dating can be summarized under the heading "self-awareness with open communication." There are ways to plan ahead to take the same approach in long-term relationships.

PREVENTION STRATEGY 1: Cultivate self-awareness with open communication

"I don't know if it's my disorder or my personality, but I tend to be very reactive to people. One word or even a look can set me off. When I argue with Mandy [wife], I have to be aware of my overreactions to her tone of voice, which can sound like an annoyed babysitter. There's like this drone in my head: 'She doesn't love me,' 'I'm a burden to her and the kids, and all that.' Then when she says something that sounds negative or demeaning, I just start spiraling.

"When this happens I take some time by myself and regroup and look at the thoughts I'm having so that I don't just say something horrible. My therapist says I'm learning 'emotional regulation skills,' but I just call it chillin'.

"But that's not the end of it—we come back together later so I can tell her what was going on with me, that it wasn't all her fault, that I wasn't just being mean. She tells me what she heard me say, and I'm surprised at how she hears things totally differently than I meant them. These conversations really have helped our relationship; she's learning not to take things so hard, and I'm learning that having bipolar disorder doesn't mean I can just say and do whatever I want."

—Sylvie, a 35-year-old with bipolar II disorder

As the quote shows, relationship harmony is owning your own emotional reactions and being sensitive to your partner's. Although extreme, Sylvie's emotional reactions were often valid. Mandy was well-intentioned but tended to talk to Sylvie like she was a child. Her tone became a trigger for Sylvie and made her react strongly to even single words or gestures.

Let's briefly review the communication skills described in Chapter 7. In the midst of an argument, a statement of active listening like "You're feeling really angry at me right now because you think I'm just doing this to be mean" can make your partner feel understood. You can also make a positive request: "I'd appreciate having some time to chill by myself and figure out why I'm getting so upset. Then we can talk about it later when I've calmed down. OK with you?" or "I'm having a hard time hearing you right now. Can you please try to use a tone you'd use when talking to me as an adult?" Rehearsing these requests with your partner when you're not excessively angry can make it easier to say them in the heat of the moment.

PREVENTION STRATEGY 2: Evaluate the role your partner takes in your care

When you are ill and in the hospital, you might see the best from your partner. Hopefully, your partner understands that BD is an illness like any other and that, following an episode, you need more than the usual amount of support, compassion, and understanding. In contrast, when you are between episodes you may still be emotionally volatile, which they may have more trouble understanding.

After a mood episode, some partners unequivocally devote themselves to making sure their partner with BD is healthy, whether this intervention is wanted or not. We call this the "lawnmower partner": someone who gets out in front of you and tries to mow down any obstacles that could cause you stress or contribute to a recurrence. This is a difficult responsibility for a partner to take on, and inevitably they will get exhausted and frustrated and you will find it intrusive. It's important to encourage your partner to engage in adequate self-care, whether that means spending time with their friends, getting regular exercise, or getting their own therapy.

You can also help them revise their caregiving role by prioritizing your own care. On a concrete level, this means filling your prescriptions without being asked, keeping to a regular sleeping and eating schedule, making your own medical appointments, and avoiding alcohol and street drugs. You can set limits with your partner by saying, "I appreciate all the help you want to give me, and I know it comes out of compassion. But I do best when I take care of my own health." Encourage them to treat you like an equal partner rather than a patient with a series of problems to be solved.

PREVENTION STRATEGY 3: Ease back into a routine

The interval following a mood episode—especially one that required hospitalization or intensive outpatient treatment—may require getting reacquainted with your partner and your previous lifestyle, much like returning from a long trip. Anxiety about being close during this interval is a natural part of coping with BD as a couple. The key strategy is to move slowly and not expect much from each other during this recovery phase. Activities you both enjoyed previously, such as sports, should be revisited gradually. You may not want (or be able) to interact with other couples just yet.

PREVENTION STRATEGY 4: Rediscover sexual intimacy

It is common in any long-term relationship to go in and out of periods of being sexually active with your mate. Numerous books have been written on this subject, most famously *The Joy of Sex* (Comfort, 2013). It's especially hard to jump right back into a sexual relationship when you've just been depressed. Your self-esteem has probably taken a hit and you may feel uncomfortable with your body, all of which make it hard to relax. If you worry that you are no longer attracted to your mate or have lost your sex drive altogether, here are some actions to take:

STRATEGY 4A: Ask yourself whether it's the depression talking

If you have other symptoms of depression—insomnia, loss of interests, fatigue, sadness—it's likely that you also have "loss of libido." Physical exercise can help reignite your sex drive, in part because your mood will improve and in part because you will feel better about your body.

STRATEGY 4B: Discuss with your doctor whether medication dosages can be adjusted or other medications substituted

Antidepressants and some mood stabilizers are associated with decreased sex drive or performance. However, it won't always be clear whether your decreased drive is due to unresolved depressive symptoms or the medications used to treat them. With your psychiatrist, you may want to examine the timing of your decreased libido in relation to when you started the relevant medication.

STRATEGY 4C: If you suspect other physical causes of your loss of desire, ask your doctor whether hormonal tests would be informative: testosterone for men, estrogen for women

Changes in hormones are a feature of aging, and can be especially tough for women during menopause. Hormonal supplements are an option, but they can have side effects that require further discussion.

STRATEGY 4D: Rediscover your sexual relationship gradually

Get to know your partner again through touch, massages, hugging, and other gradual steps toward intimacy before attempting intercourse.

STRATEGY 4E: If you are not feeling sexual toward your partner but are sexually attracted to others, it may be time to try some couple therapy

Loss of intimacy can occur when one person feels "one-down" in a partnership, or no longer trusts their partner. If your partner has had an affair with someone else, you are particularly likely to feel that way, as will your partner if you have had an affair during a manic episode.

Solving Daily Relationship Problems

People with BD experience the same couple conflicts about everyday matters that all couples experience, but these get exaggerated in intensity after an episode. Problems related to household management (cooking, cleaning, shopping, and so on), taking care of kids, finances, in-laws, and pets come to the fore. As you recover, your spouse may expect more and more of you, and you may be eager to resume roles that were put on hold while you were ill. However, the pace of your partner's expectations and your ability to meet them may not match up.

Many partners do not know that major depressive episodes can require an average of 6 months to lift, or that moods may improve before one's level of cognitive functioning resumes. So, your partner may be demanding a level of performance that you are not up to yet. At times you may need to push yourself to do things you really don't feel up to doing (driving your kids to soccer early in the morning; spending parts of the weekend cleaning), but it is important to pace yourself and encourage patience from your spouse.

IN-THE-MOMENT STRATEGY: Discuss collaborative problem solving

Other couple problems may be amenable to in-the-moment solutions through collaborative problem solving, as shown in the worksheet on page 144. Simple problems (such as who will take out the trash) usually don't require this level of complex problem solving. The difficulties that cause significant couple conflicts tend to be emotional rather than practical (for example, "who takes out the trash" may be one indicator of a larger problem, such as "both partners feel like their time is not respected by the other partner"). If a problem seems too big to submit to the steps in the worksheet, try to break it down into smaller units and solve each unit individually, so that disagreements don't become bigger than they have to be. When you and your partner can solve one little part of a problem, there will be more of a sense of collaboration in tackling others. In this section you'll read an example of in-the-moment problem solving.

An Example of Collaborative Problem Solving

Karla, age 39, was recovering from a lengthy bipolar II depressive episode. The recovery process had taken longer than she or her husband, Justin, expected, with many twists and turns. Justin had been reasonably patient, but his mother, Isabel, had been making comments such as "When is she going to get better?" and, within earshot of the couple's two children, "Do you think she's trying hard enough?" Justin and his mother were close, and Isabel was also close with the kids.

Karla and Justin had learned the collaborative problem-solving method in couple sessions, but their definitions of this problem differed. Karla was angry that Justin didn't rush to her defense, whereas Justin felt that Karla was overreacting to

COLLABORATIVE
PROBLEM-SOLVING WORKSHEET

What is the problem? Define it from both partners' perspectives.

Brainstorm solutions: Throw out every possible solution, even ones that may seem unfeasible or silly. Don't squash any options just yet.

Evaluate the pros and cons of each proposed solution.

Solution number	Advantages	Disadvantages
_____	_____	_____
	_____	_____
_____	_____	_____
	_____	_____

Choose one solution or set of solutions:

Develop an implementation plan: Who will do what?

Revisit the initial problem later: Was it solved? If not, why not? Go back to the beginning. Was it defined correctly? Were the solutions feasible?

questions that any reasonable person would ask. Their proposed solutions varied from "Justin shouldn't talk to his mother about Karla anymore" to "Karla should defend herself when Isabel says something about her disorder." After weighing the pros and cons of each solution, they homed in on the only solution that involved actions on both of their parts: When Isabel raised questions about Karla's progress, Karla would nondefensively tell her about her medications and exercise plan. Then Justin would talk to Isabel privately about not bringing up such issues around Karla, and offer a progress report now and again.

The solution did not work well. When they tried to implement it the following Saturday evening, Justin's mother temporarily withheld comments but, later in the evening over dinner, said, "I heard an NPR [National Public Radio] program about bipolar disorder, and they said you should try a new medication called Latrigine or Lamuda or something." When this occurred, Karla burst into tears and ran out of the room.

Karla and Justin talked this over several times and engaged their therapist in the process. They concluded that Justin needed to be more assertive with his mother about bringing up Karla's health, in whatever form. They also agreed that Karla's residual depression was coloring how she interpreted Isabel's interventions, and that part of the plan necessitated her letting certain comments go. A more comprehensive solution followed, in which Justin spoke at length with his mother about why Karla was getting hurt, and Karla rehearsed a limit-setting response to Isabel ("I don't want to get into that right now; that's a sensitive subject for me"). They also agreed that dinners at their house involving Isabel might not be such a good idea until Karla had fully recovered and that Karla should express a willingness to interact with Isabel in other settings, particularly when their children were involved.

The solution eventually worked, with some additional tweaks. Most importantly, Karla and Justin felt they had solved the problem collaboratively. Karla realized that part of her depression was related to the stigma of her disorder and how it was being expressed within their family, as well as her own self-criticism about her progress.

Taking Stock

All illnesses put stress on relationships, but in BD, relationship stress can contribute to mood episodes, and mood episodes can contribute to relationship stress. Nonetheless, people with BD are just as able as anyone to have intimate, long-term relationships or marriages despite emotional upheavals.

Depending on where you are in your romantic life—dating, in a new or long-lasting relationship, or staying single—review the skills discussed in this chapter and include them in your relapse prevention plans (Chapters 1 and 2). Strong partnerships can be of considerable value in supporting you when you are at risk for developing mania or depression or when recovering from either. They can also help you deal with conflicts that arise with your family of origin. Your willingness to work with your partner to improve communication and solve problems will almost certainly contribute to the longevity of the relationship.

9

making the best use of your skills at work and school

Problems with functioning at school and work are quite common in BD, but the nature of these difficulties varies considerably from person to person. You may be working but find that it takes significantly more effort than it used to. You may have made good progress in college or in a vocational program, but an episode of mania or depression set you back for a full semester or even a year. Maybe you love your job, but disturbances in memory, attention, and concentration have made it hard to function at your best. Alternatively, you may have lost your job (or left school) because you became depressed when work demands got overwhelming. If you've experienced any of these problems, you are certainly not alone—about 65% of people with BD have unstable employment. The factors associated with employment instability include ongoing depressive symptoms; physical illnesses; cognitive problems, such as impaired memory or processing speed; and disruptive life events.

Whatever your situation, you have every right to expect satisfaction in the working world or while getting an education. School and work impose different kinds of demands, but the challenges that BD presents in the two settings are similar. The good news is that there are a number of "hacks" or workarounds you can use to succeed.

Disclosing Your BD

 "I'm afraid I'll get a bad reaction to telling people at work/school that I have bipolar disorder."

If you've just gotten a job or started college (or a vocational training program), should you disclose your disorder and to whom? The issues here are more complex than those involved in dating (see Chapter 8), but the same problems with stigma apply. We know that employers are guarded about hiring people with psychiatric disorders, often because of misguided assumptions about violence or potential disability.

Because of the Americans with Disabilities Act (1990; *www.ada.gov*), prospective employers are not allowed to ask on a hiring form or in an interview whether you have a mental health condition. They cannot fire you, refuse to promote you, or make you leave simply because you have a diagnosis. Similarly, if you want to further your education by taking vocational, college, or graduate-level courses, the educational institution cannot refuse to admit you or advance you because of your diagnosis.

In job settings, the rub is this: Some jobs do require disclosure of mental health conditions and are not in violation of the Disabilities Act, such as government-regulated jobs or jobs with high levels of physical and mental endurance requirements. For example, if you're taking lithium and experiencing hand tremors, you may not be eligible for a job that requires steady hands to operate a mechanical saw. Nonetheless, the employer would have to prove that the disorder will interfere with your job functions and that no on-the-job accommodations can be made.

PREVENTION STRATEGY 1: Evaluate the pros and cons of disclosing

There are clearly advantages to disclosing your disorder in a new job. Doing so will enable you to work with your supervisor (or the HR department) to obtain *reasonable accommodations* (see below). It may increase your own acceptance of the disorder when coworkers turn out to be more accepting than you expected. On the practical side, when people at work know about your disorder, they may be able to help you should you have a suicidal crisis, a panic attack, or an overwhelming desire to punch your boss.

The disadvantages are fairly straightforward: Employers who hold stigmatizing attitudes could decide to fire you or cut your hours. This is illegal, of course, and the business could come under fire from the U.S. Equal Employment Opportunity Commission, but proving legally that you were fired because of your disorder is difficult.

Some of my patients have told me that once the word gets out at work, their behavior is interpreted in terms of the diagnostic label. If they get annoyed at someone or something, their response is viewed as "over the top." If they are working extremely hard to meet a deadline, others wonder if they've become manic. These situations can cause varying levels of discomfort, and can be a deal-breaker (necessitating finding another job) for some. There are also generational differences: millennials (those born from the early 1980s to the early 2000s) appear to be more comfortable making disclosures about psychiatric problems than those in earlier generations.

If you've been at a job for a number of months and haven't told your employer or coworkers, you probably have good reasons for being cautious. However, you may have a good idea of who among your colleagues can be trusted with this kind of information. If you're considering telling a close friend at work, how have they talked about mental health in the past? Do they tend to gossip about any of your colleagues? Do they treat people with respect and confidentiality?

As for disclosing at school, the advantages and disadvantages are similar. The Individuals with Disabilities Education Act and Section 504 of the Rehabilitation Act provide protections for young adults (up to age 21) with mental illness in educational settings, and the Americans with Disabilities Act provides protections for adults. Schools cannot refuse to give you an appropriate education because of a documented physical or mental disability. You can read up on these laws at *https://sites.ed.gov/idea* or *www.ada.gov.*

When deciding whether to disclose, consider a couple of issues. First, why do you want your employer or teacher/professor to know? Is it because you want work or school accommodations? Is it because others have disclosed their mental health problems and gotten a good response from colleagues? Are you looking for emotional support? These are all good reasons, but they need to be balanced against the negative backlash that could occur in your setting. **My recommendation is the same one I'd give for any health condition: Keep it private unless you want something specific—such as an accommodation in your work hours, working conditions, or classroom assignments—to come out of the disclosure.**

 "I want to disclose my disorder but have no idea what or how much to say."

As was true for dating, people vary in how much they disclose to current or potential employers or teachers. Some tell their whole story to every new acquaintance, including the hospitalizations, the negative experiences with psychiatrists and therapists, the failed medication trials, and their residential care. Others give just a brief outline: when they were first diagnosed, what medications they take, and whether they see a therapist. Here is a compromise way to broach the topic with an employer (or an instructor or professor):

> "I am dealing with some issues with my mood and energy levels. These are problems that have a biological basis, but it means that my work may be irregular at times. I may have a lot of energy and get lots done some of the time, and at other times I may seem slowed down or low in motivation. I'd like your help in arranging [my work hours, whether I work at home some of the time, and so on]. I'd like to get regular feedback about how I'm doing so I can meet my responsibilities."

In this example there is no mention of BD. You may prefer to give it a name (and the employer or professor may have already apprehended it), but it may not be necessary as long as they understand what accommodations you're asking for.

PREVENTION STRATEGY 2: Ask for reasonable accommodations

The best reason to disclose your disorder is to ask for adjustments to the job duties, context, setting, or hours to fit the limits imposed by your moods or sleep patterns. Good accommodations will make job tasks less stressful, more comfortable, and often less time-consuming so that you can perform at your best level.

My experience has been that people with BD perform best in jobs (or in educational settings) that have some or all of the following accommodations. The list is not exhaustive, nor should you expect any employer or school registrar to meet all of them:

- Consistent and predictable (rather than constantly variable) hours, allowing you to have a regular sleep and wake schedule
- A somewhat late start to the workday or school day (for example, starting at 10 A.M. if it's supposed to start at 8 or 9 A.M.) to help you deal with sleep inertia
- The freedom to schedule doctor or therapist appointments without having to sacrifice pay or be denied school credits

- Physical distance from other workers or students and enough breaks to allow you to decompress
- Written feedback from supervisors or teachers with suggestions for improving your performance, rather than only oral feedback that may be emotionally triggering.

When applying for jobs, you may want to ask for accommodations after you've been offered the job (and before you accept) so that your request is not used to exclude you from employment. Alternatively, you may want to work at the job for a couple of weeks before coming in with a list of accommodations, because you may not know what to ask for yet (for example, you didn't realize you would be working in a noisy room and could benefit from noise-canceling headphones or a white noise machine). In larger companies, the HR department may be able to coach you on what accommodations would work for you and the company.

Imagine that first thing in the morning you are asked to balance the books on yesterday's sales. It may be far easier for you to do this later in the day, once you're fully awake. If the business allows flexibility on this task, your request for a later deadline may be eminently reasonable. Or let's say you're working with a therapist you really like but their only available appointment is on Tuesday at 2:00, right in the middle of the workday. You should be able to negotiate a late lunch (or a longer lunch) on Tuesday. Some employers get sticky about the number of hours you put in, so if necessary, you could offer to stay an hour longer that day.

Of course, for certain accommodations you may have to disclose your disorder. Be wary of any employer or HR department that offers you a position and, when you ask for an accommodation, says, "You should have told us about that earlier." You are not obligated to tell anyone about your illness when you are applying for a job. If you believe you've been mistreated, contact your local chapter of the U.S. Equal Employment Opportunity Commission (*www.eeoc.gov* or call 800-669-4000).

PREVENTION STRATEGY 3: If you're in school, consult with the Student Disabilities Office

Although you may bristle at the idea of calling BD a disability, this is a catch-all term schools use for anything that could inhibit progress. A documented disability (one that a doctor has verified) can protect you if your symptoms interfere with your attendance or coursework. Some professors like to be tough guys and insist that everyone have the same deadlines, but staff from the disabilities office can intervene on your behalf to help you arrange for different requirements. School accommodations may include getting an extension on a paper, avoiding taking tests early in the morning, or arranging make-up exams if the timing of an exam interferes with your treatment. Those simple adjustments can make a world of difference when you are depressed.

Strategies for Success at School and Work

 "I really want to be effective, but it's hard to do that when my symptoms interfere."

To what extent has depression interfered with finishing up your courses at school or completing your assignments at work? Symptoms of depression and anxiety can make it extra hard to get to school or work on time, complete the full day, or focus on one task at a time. The apathy and anhedonia (lack of experiencing pleasure) that are a part of depression may contribute to low motivation. You may have experienced the opposite during periods of hypomania or mania: feeling that other people are moving too slowly or getting frustrated at others' lack of progress.

PREVENTION STRATEGY 1: Go to school or work part-time

This strategy can be especially helpful when you are coming off of a mood episode. Many college students go through depressive episodes in the fall semester and are not fully recovered by the spring. Most colleges have academic advisors or counselors who can guide you on what courses to take in the spring to ease back into the college environment.

If you have had to take time off from school or your job, you may be tempted to come back with "all guns blazing" and take on much more work than you can handle. This plan usually backfires because of the cognitive limitations that go along with depression or mania/hypomania (see below). Choose a less demanding course schedule than would be typical of you (or the school you attend). Going back to school half-time may be a reasonable way to balance your work hours with leisure time and regular sleep. You may take longer than your peers to finish college, but in the short term a lighter workload will increase your chances of succeeding in school with your health intact. When coming off of an episode, consider working part-time if that is feasible. Even if part-time isn't affordable for long, it can be less expensive in the long run than compromising your health to work full-time and then having to quit.

"I get anxious and overwhelmed at work (or school) when I have too much to do. Then I get defensive or irritable with my coworkers. How do I manage this?"

This is one area where in-the-moment strategies will be of greatest help. If you're working with a deadline, and everyone around you is rushing around making demands, your stress and anxiety may become intolerable. In addition to the strategies below, Chapter 3 describes a number of stress-reduction methods, some of which can be applied during your workday.

IN-THE-MOMENT STRATEGY 1: Start the day with a brief meditation exercise

Meditating may relax you. A 20- to 30-minute sitting and breathing meditation or a body scan (*www.headspace.com/meditation/body-scan*) can help focus your attention as you start to deal with the day's assignments.

IN-THE-MOMENT STRATEGY 2: Take short but frequent breaks

This strategy may need to be negotiated in advance with your supervisor, but you may prefer 10-minute breaks every hour to 30-minute breaks every 3 hours. If you feel overstimulated by other people, and especially if you feel like snapping at them, find a quiet place to sit by yourself. If you find it hard to just sit and breathe, use the distractions that help you relax when you're at home: Watch some music videos, read, work on a puzzle, or play a video game.

IN-THE-MOMENT STRATEGY 3: Talk to a friend or coworker

A brief conversation with a trusted friend outside of the workplace or school environment—one who understands you and values your privacy—may be just the ticket during a stressful work interval. A coworker may assume you want advice on handling your assignments, which may add to your stress when you prefer to talk to someone who will just listen. Unfortunately, in the middle of the workday and without a scheduled appointment, therapists are not usually of much help.

IN-THE-MOMENT STRATEGY 4: Ask to continue your work at home

Since the COVID pandemic, more and more employers allow employees to do some or all of their work remotely. Discuss the workplace policy with your supervisor. If you are expected to produce a written report by day's end, your supervisor may not care where you do it as long as you get it done. Taking it home may make a world of difference to you in the moment.

IN-THE-MOMENT STRATEGY 5: Know your stress limits

Certain jobs (such as nursing, construction, retail, or restaurant service) may require being at a certain location throughout the day, and may come with frequent or unexpected requests to work additional shifts. If you consistently find that you're getting stressed out by work, be extra cautious about how many tasks and work shifts you're taking on.

Some people keep in their mind the image of a stress thermometer (see page 155) to depict where they are on a 0–100 scale of emotional and physiological stress. You may find that as you approach the highest levels, you feel sweaty, your heart pounds, and your breathing becomes quick or labored. Your mood may change from mild annoyance to anger or even rage. If you find that the scale matches up to how you experience stress, pick a point on the scale (50–60 is typical) where switching to another activity (or leaving work, or not taking an additional shift) will allow you to avoid a meltdown or a major confrontation. Again, accommodations that allow for breaks in the work routine can often be arranged in advance.

If you're consistently finding your job too stressful or that you are on the verge of a mood recurrence, determine whether a job change is in the cards. I don't say this lightly; jobs are hard to find, and you may have worked hard to find this one, but don't stay in a job that poses a threat to your health.

 "Problems with memory and attention are interfering with my work/school performance."

If you've experienced problems with your memory, attention, or concentration on the job, you're in good company. Many people with BD—about 40% by some estimates—experience ongoing cognitive problems even when not in a symptomatic state. Cognitive problems can be very discouraging when you've already been through a lengthy episode and are trying to resume a semblance of a normal lifestyle.

When people are depressed, short-term memory can be impaired, which usually shows up as forgetting people's names or telephone numbers (when they've just told them to you), making calculations, or reading. Concentration can be especially difficult. Some people also forget the steps required to complete tasks (for example, the forms you have to fill out to get paid every month). Some people describe "brain

STRESS THERMOMETER

Things that have stressed you out lately:

_____

_____

_____

_____

Make a 0–100 rating of the most distressed or angry you were today.

Things you did (or can do) to make yourself feel better:

100 — Enraged	STOP! _____ _____
Angry	Calm down _____ _____
60 — Upset	Relax _____ _____
Sad	Think about what really works _____ _____
40 — Happy	Think about something good _____ _____
Very happy	
0 —	Do something that boosts your mood* _____ _____

*See the box on page 25 for ideas.

fog," especially in the morning—the inability to focus on tasks and tune out irrelevant information, retrieve words, recall events, and focus on conversations.

Mania or hypomania can also be associated with problems with concentrating, confusion, and forgetfulness, either during or after the episode. One study found that the low-level depressive symptoms that persist after a manic episode are associated with delays in regaining the level of work, school, or social functioning one had before the manic episode.

PREVENTION STRATEGY 1: Reevaluate your medication regimen with your doctor

If you've been struggling with memory or attention at work, arrange an appointment with your doctor to discuss your medications and dosages. Some of your medications may be contributing to memory loss—for example, lithium, despite its excellent record in relapse prevention, has the side effect of impaired memory. Are your doses too high, such that they are interfering with your mental sharpness in the morning, making you feel sedated? You may be a candidate for one of the cognitive-enhancing medications like modafinil.

When discovering that their medications make it hard to remember or process information, some people immediately jump to quitting their medications. **It's important to explore getting your meds adjusted before you decide to stop taking them.** Stopping medications like lithium, especially if you do so abruptly, can bring on a severe recurrence and contribute to feeling suicidal (see also Chapter 13).

PREVENTION STRATEGY 2: Try to exercise regularly

There is some mixed evidence that regular exercise improves cognitive functioning; its most reliable benefits appear to be on mood (see Chapter 10). A good plan is to aim to be physically active for 20–30 minutes at least 4 days a week. Physical activity is not necessarily going to the gym; it can be briskly walking the dog, dancing, or riding your bike to work.

PREVENTION STRATEGY 3: Avoid alcohol and cannabis

You may look forward to having a drink or smoking a joint after work or school, and occasional use may not be harmful. Although alcohol and marijuana can temporarily lift your mood or decrease your anxiety, they can make memory loss worse over time. Regular use will interfere with the effectiveness of your medications, increasing your chances of a recurrence. A glass of wine with dinner may be OK, but avoid hitting the bar or pub immediately after work or selecting activities that require alcohol. Managing substance abuse is a whole subject in itself, as you'll see in Chapter 12.

PREVENTION STRATEGY 4: Play online computer games

Think of your memory and attention as muscles that get stronger with more use. Video gaming can help keep your thinking sharper, as long as you play games that require some problem solving, memory, or puzzles (a good overall website is *www.brainhq.com*). Lumosity (*www.lumosity.com/en*) has a number of online exercises that appear to have benefits for cognitive functioning.

PREVENTION STRATEGY 5: Look into cognitive rehabilitation

If available in your community, enroll in a cognitive rehabilitation program that meets at least weekly and takes you through guided strategies for attention, concentration, and memory. Your doctor may need to refer you to one of these. There are also cognitive exercises you can do at home that are similar to those you might do in therapy (for example, *https://worksheets.happyneuronpro.com/packets*), but cognitive rehab, much like physical therapy, is more likely to benefit you if there is a clinician or a group working alongside of you.

PREVENTION STRATEGY 6: Avoid excessive sugar

Diet is the focus of Chapter 11, as there is now mounting evidence that proper diets can improve mood and cognition. For now, just consider your intake of sugar. People with a daily habit of drinking sugary beverages—such as Pepsi or Coke, Red Bull, or various fruit juices including Gatorade—may be more likely to have memory impairments and smaller brain volumes. The good news is that you can reverse this damage by following a low-glycemic, low-sugar diet, such as keto or Mediterranean.

IN-THE-MOMENT STRATEGY 1: Use automated reminders

If you frequently forget meetings, classes, callbacks, or little things that need to be done alongside bigger-ticket items, use the notifications on your phone or email or keep an online task diary (for example, Microsoft Outlook has a separate task list that can be paired with your daily schedule). As annoying as they may be, voice assistants like Siri or Alexa can be programmed to remind you of these tasks.

IN-THE-MOMENT STRATEGY 2: Keep a log of what you're doing throughout the day and the steps required to complete each task

The act of writing down the steps can enhance your recall of them later.

IN-THE-MOMENT STRATEGY 3: Record your distractions

If you get distracted, keep sticky notes around and jot down what distracted you. Then go back to what you're doing. If the same sounds or conversations distract you, you may need to alter your work environment. For example, at this very moment, I am trying to avoid being distracted by the sounds of leaf blowers and trucks backing up. Listening to music on earbuds can help drown out background noise, but other people's music, especially if played loudly, can be highly distracting (see Chapter 4 for suggestions on how to handle this situation).

Social media can be a major source of distraction and, in fact, it's designed to do just that. If you often scroll to your social media pages while at work or in school, use a timer, with the self-guided instruction to work on a given task for X minutes without giving in to distraction.

IN-THE-MOMENT STRATEGY 4: Take meditation breaks

There is some evidence that meditation is associated with enhanced memory and relaxation. On a 10-minute work or school break you can do a 5-minute meditation, perhaps with the aid of a prerecorded exercise (such as *www.youtube.com/watch?v=i50ZAs7v9es*).

When You Need a Break from Work after an Episode

If you currently have a job but are having trouble completing tasks, consider whether any of the accommodations listed earlier would be an effective temporary fix. But if you have been having consistent problems keeping a job because of ongoing periods of depression or cognitive impairment, consider applying for Social Security Disability Insurance (SSDI) payments. Applying for SSDI should not be a source of shame or equated with giving up. It may be an essential step that removes a major stressor when you are coming off of a mood episode.

PREVENTION STRATEGY 1: Apply for disability through your employer

You may be paying insurance premiums for short- or long-term disability and, with the appropriate medical evaluation, may be eligible for disability payments. The other way is to apply for SSDI from the federal government, which has to be done through a local Social Security office in your city. It may help to consult a social worker or vocation rehabilitation counselor who will help you get the documentation you need. Keep in mind that getting disability payments can take up to 6 months, so this is not the step to take in emergency situations (like needing money immediately).

A question may be how long you want to be on disability: Just until the end of this mood episode? The rest of the calendar year? An indefinite period? It can be harder to get back into the workforce if you are on disability for a long period of time.

PREVENTION STRATEGY 2: Use your time to build skills and volunteer

It is important to use your strengths and build skills in anticipation of returning to the job market. If you think you would like a career in journalism, volunteer at a local newspaper. Working in the health care industry? There are many hospitals, nursing homes, and residential facilities that regularly take volunteers, sometimes for positions with many responsibilities. Animal care? Consider working at the Humane Society. Music? Volunteer as an usher at a rock 'n' roll or jazz festival.

You may find the volunteer work more meaningful than what you experienced in your paid work, without all of the pressure. Many people are surprised to find that their volunteer jobs, which may have been started just to fill time, end up satisfying an important drive for meaning that can be carried into paid opportunities.

Taking Stock

After reading this chapter, think of what your options are and try filling out the planning sheet on page 160. Its purpose is not necessarily to lock you into a specific plan of action but to consider your options. You may answer these questions differently when you're in the midst of a depressive episode compared to when you're feeling OK but aren't satisfied with your line of work.

WORK AND SCHOOL PLANNING SHEET

I am reentering the job market (or going to school) after a mood episode. What "reasonable accommodations" should I ask for?

Would I want to disclose having bipolar disorder, and what would I say?

If I am feeling depressed and having a tough time getting through the workday or school day, what can I do?

What strategies can help me with anxiety or stress on the job?

What strategies for improving memory and attention can I use?

What are the arguments for or against applying for disability?

If you are having trouble finding jobs for which you are qualified, consult an occupational therapist or a "life coach." They can help you evaluate whether your current employment is a good fit or what other options may be available (*www.betterup.com/en/about-us* and *https://coachconnect.life/life-coaching-services*).

Finally, don't lose hope! Accepting the limitations imposed by your disorder is not easy. BD can delay but it will not erase your life goals. Talk to others who have the disorder and see how they've handled similar situations. Many highly talented, creative, and productive people have had this disorder, as recounted in Kay Jamison's book *Touched with Fire: Manic-Depressive Illness and the Artistic Temperament* (1993).

10

staying healthy

PHYSICAL ACTIVITY

A big question on the minds of many people with BD is how to stay physically healthy, despite the low energy and diminished motivation of depression, the intense food cravings (or lack of appetite), the physical and emotional pain, and the medications that can cause weight gain. When manic or hypomanic, some people with BD feel driven to be constantly physically active to the point of exhaustion. Then, when they're depressed, they give up activity entirely.

Physical activity and a healthy diet have long been known to improve mood, cognition, learning, and memory. They can help you manage cardiovascular risk factors, such as weight, blood pressure, kidney functioning, and insulin sensitivity. They are important in protecting you from mood episodes and helping speed up recovery from them. Chapter 11 offers strategies for maintaining a healthy diet. This chapter offers strategies for healthy physical activity. I use the term *physical activity* broadly to mean anything that requires moving your muscles. Most people equate it with focused, structured exercise routines, but physical activity takes many different forms: walking the dog, going up and down stairs, gardening, riding a bike to work, or just walking from place to place rather than driving. Although we know that increasing physical activity is a genuinely helpful health habit, we know relatively little about what kind or intensity is helpful when you're living with BD, how to make it work when you're depressed and lacking in motivation, or how much is too much when you're manic or hypomanic.

The Love–Hate Relationship between BD and Physical Activity

"My doctor and I are good at two-way communication. When I get depressed, he tells me to start exercising. And when he tells me to start exercising, I tell him to go _____ himself."

—*42-year-old woman with bipolar II disorder*

You may have heard well-intentioned but self-evident recommendations from doctors or family members about being physically active and following a healthy diet, as if doing so were just a question of joining a gym or stocking your shelves. This kind of advice can feel very invalidating. Indeed, people don't usually adopt healthy lifestyles just because other people tell them they should. More often, they make changes when these changes give them a sense of control over their lives.

There are a lot of good reasons to be physically active other than just to lose weight. In fact, people experience benefits from physical activity even when their weight doesn't change at all: Their mood improves, they have more energy, more sexual drive, a more positive attitude toward life, and may be able to get by on fewer medications or lower doses. Nonetheless, as mentioned in prior chapters, during depression you may have a diminished capacity to experience pleasure or rewards (anhedonia), whether those rewards are physical, social, or material. Anhedonia can interfere with your motivation and diminish any joy you might experience from physical activity. As a result, exercise is a bigger challenge for people with BD than for many others. This is among the reasons that messages like "You should just go out and exercise" feel invalidating or lacking in empathy.

PREVENTION STRATEGY: Find out how your current level of physical activity is affecting your mood

As has been true throughout this book, the first step in changing health behaviors is to track what you're doing now and how it relates to your mood. Keeping records of your baseline level of activity will help you determine how much more or less you need to do and how to achieve a balance. Using the weekly Physical Activity and Diet log on page 165, start by recording your current activity level for each day of the week (such as, how many minutes you are moving your body in some way) and a daily rating of your mood (a 1–10 rating of depression or a scale of –5 [*depressed*] to +5 [*manic*] may be most familiar). If your physical activity occurs during a discrete period during the day, you can make a mood rating before this period and one after it. For now, don't worry about your diet; I'll ask you to fill in that part of the log in Chapter 11. Keeping these records over several weeks or months will begin to clarify whether physical activity and diet are contributing to your mood stability or changes, as well as how often an increase in your activity goes along with healthier eating.

 "I don't exercise when I'm depressed—I can't make myself do it. How do I talk myself into it?"

PREVENTION STRATEGY 1: Define your personal health goals

We've all had the experience of deciding one night to launch an intensive exercise program the next day, involving running, swimming, weight training, or bicycling. Then the next morning comes around and doing any of these things seems about as likely as hiking up Mt. Kilimanjaro.

When you're depressed, and sometimes even when not, being told "You need to exercise more" is about as inviting as "Plan your next five dental appointments." The word *exercise* can in itself be triggering, bringing up difficult memories and negative self-talk. Because it's always so highly recommended, people with BD feel pushed too hard, which backfires. Instead, think about your *quality of life* as the broader objective: your feeling of well-being in the context of your goals, expectations, and the culture around you. Physical activity is only one element that contributes to quality of life.

- **Step 1: Motivate yourself to exercise based on your immediate life goals.** What is most important to you right now? What would you like to be able to say 6–12 months from now that would feel like progress? The following are examples of how people often answer these questions; check off any answers that apply to you. Some people write these life goals on a sheet of paper and hang it in places where they'll see it every day; others would rather not have to constantly look at it:

  ❑ Alleviating my depression without causing a switch into mania or hypomania
  ❑ Losing weight and feeling healthier
  ❑ Having a healthy romantic relationship
  ❑ Feeling less stressed out and anxious in work or in classes
  ❑ Reducing the number of medications I take
  ❑ Sleeping better
  ❑ Other (specify _____)

PHYSICAL ACTIVITY AND DIET CHART

For each day, record what you ate at each meal, amount of time spent exercising, mood, and wake/bedtimes.

Day	Breakfast	Lunch	Dinner	Snacks	Drinks	Physical activity (~ time)	Mood for the day (–5 to +5)	Wake time	Bedtime
Monday									
Tuesday									
Wednesday									
Thursday									
Friday									
Saturday									
Sunday									

• **Step 2: Consider the relevance of physical activity to these goals.** Your goals for exercising may be quite different when you're feeling OK than when you're depressed, and the exercise plans will differ correspondingly. If your main goal is to get out of your current state of depression, then exercising (even moderately) will be one of many things that can help, assuming it is not so severe as to make physical activity feel impossible. If your main goal is to meet someone new and have a romantic relationship, then losing weight and being in shape is likely to be important to you. If your main goal is feeling less stressed at school, physical activity may play a smaller role in your daily activities but will almost certainly help with your attention and concentration. Getting exercise may improve your blood pressure, which may mean you can get off one or more sedating hypertensive medications.

In planning an exercise routine, it's best to keep your eye on personal goals, such as better moods, less stress, or better sleep. Try to shift your focus away from immediate and concrete goals like "number of calories consumed" or "number of steps walked each day." It's fairly easy to set concrete goals when you're feeling OK, but when you get depressed, you'll wonder why you ever set those goals. Set more positive personal objectives, like feeling more energy or more confidence about yourself or being less stressed out.

PREVENTION STRATEGY 2: Make exercise work for you

If you've tried to exercise before but it hasn't worked, how would you like to do it differently now? Several principles can help you engage in an exercise routine.

STRATEGY 2A: If you haven't exercised in quite some time, start with a very easy exercise—a walk around the block, some jumping jacks, a mild yoga routine

Think more about *physical activity* than exercise, with the goal being to just make more physical movements. You can be in your pajamas; you don't have to go to a gym. You will probably see mood improvement quickly, but avoid being self-critical if you can't do it every day or if you find the activities painful. If you have had recent health problems, a quick consult with your general practitioner (GP) may help you define what is possible or advisable right now.

STRATEGY 2B: Develop the routine when you're feeling reasonably well and try to make it a habit

Use the "start low, go slow" approach: begin with physical activity that almost feels too easy, but goes slightly above what you did the previous week (for example, some stretches in the morning, a walk after lunch). Then build up a week at a time, increasing the duration of physical activity to 10–15 minutes every other day, aiming for 20–30 minutes for at least 4 days of the week. If you get depressed, you may have to reduce it, but a little bit of physical activity is better than none. Don't try to initiate a full workout program when you're depressed as it may leave you feeling defeated.

STRATEGY 2C: Plan some social activities that involve physical activity and would ordinarily give you pleasure, even if they aren't that pleasurable right now

For example, going for a hike with a friend will probably be more enjoyable than going to a gym by yourself.

STRATEGY 2D: If you have usually exercised indoors, try moving it outdoors

It may sound like a cliché, but getting in touch with nature will feel rewarding even when exercising is painful.

STRATEGY 2E: Figure out a way to reward yourself for sticking to the physical activity plan

Think of things that you've been denying yourself and try to use them as incentives for meeting your activity goals. Go to see a movie in the middle of the week, go to a favorite store, get a smoothie, get into a hot tub, or call someone you haven't spoken to in a while. If you are an animal lover, a trip to the ASPCA, a local animal shelter, or the zoo will probably be rewarding. An hour of listening to music without having to do anything else is rewarding for many.

PREVENTION STRATEGY 3: Choose exercise partners with forethought

 "I find it easier to exercise with someone else, but I can't find the right person."

You don't necessarily need to have a workout buddy, but a close friend can be quite helpful when you're trying to motivate yourself. The ideal exercise partner is one who wants to just spend time with you, whether exercising or not; one who is encouraging and supportive when helping to motivate you; one who is not emotionally invested in getting you into shape; and one who won't be disappointed if you don't feel up to it that day. Exercising with a partner may be hurtful if it's a person with the wrong expectations. In my experience, friends are usually better workout buddies than family members (see section below).

If previous exercise partners have ghosted you, the thought of pairing with a new person can seem daunting. Consider the various reasons people exercise together for a while and then quit: The other person cancels too frequently, exercise takes on an overly competitive tone, one person wants to try a different sport, or one person has a chaotic or unpredictable schedule.

STRATEGY 3A: Be open about your goals

Choose a person who you feel comfortable telling about your mood swings and explain that one of the purposes is to help with your depression or anxiety (or just your personal health). Tell them that you may have to cancel or cut it short on any given day, and check whether that's OK with them.

STRATEGY 3B: Consider an exercise class

If you're finding a typical workout with that person too strenuous and they don't want to dial it back, consider enrolling in an exercise class instead (like a dance or yoga class). "Canned" online classes have the advantage that you can watch and participate in them on your own time. A "live" class may introduce you to potential exercise partners and make exercise a bit more fun.

STRATEGY 3C: Look into apps that allow you to collaborate with a stranger or a group of strangers on workouts

Good examples are Focusmate (*www.focusmate.com*), Sworkit Health (*https://sworkit.com*), and FitOn (*https://fitonapp.com*). These tend to be friendly, informal, and nonjudgmental workgroups.

STRATEGY 3D: Try a personal trainer

If you can afford a personal trainer (and hopefully not one who does double-time as a cheerleader), they may be able to help you set up a personalized plan that works within your current physical and emotional limits. You can tell them when they are pushing you too hard or expecting too much too soon. They work for you; you don't work for them!

STRATEGY 3E: Consider getting a dog

Having a dog not only guarantees you some company and warmth when you're alone, it also guarantees that you'll get a certain amount of physical activity every day. Having a dog (or another pet that needs exercise) may not work with your current work and life responsibilities but if it is an option, you'll be impressed by its effects on your mood.

PREVENTION STRATEGY 4: Go for structure and routine

 "Sometimes I exercise to exhaustion. Is this a sign of mania?"

"When I start a new exercise program, which is usually during the spring, I get like an animal coming out of hibernation. This time it began with just going to the gym early in the morning, but then I added a hike at the end of my workday. I started losing weight, and I looked and felt great. I added half an hour on the StairMaster before I went to bed, but then I couldn't sleep, and I'd get up even earlier the next day and start it all over. I can't remember when I started biking during lunch, but at some point it all ran together and I couldn't stop."
—*39-year-old woman hospitalized for mania*

Anything can be overdone. If you're exercising more than usual, feeling full of energy, and sleeping less, you're probably in a state of hypomania. Hypomania is rarely an emergency, and exercising may be a way of expending excess energy. Nonetheless, if you're exercising to an extreme, you may have to cut it back so that you don't transition into full mania. For some people, a sudden increase in physical activity from their usual state is an early warning sign of mania, much like a decreased need for sleep or rapid thoughts (see Chapter 2). If this has been true of you, include "increases in exercise" as a warning sign in your mania prevention plan, on page 41.

One way to catch this sequence early is to introduce structure into your physical activity routine. Set a limit for how much of the day you spend in heavy physical activity (for example, 90 minutes). If so, exercise from 9:00 to 10:30 A.M. each day and don't let it exceed the allotted time.

PREVENTION STRATEGY 5: Avoid working out right before bedtime

Be especially aware of how exercise can ruin the regularity of your sleep cycle, especially if you do it at night. Many people work out right before bed, thinking it will help them sleep, but it often amps them up instead. As you learned in Chapter 6, the hour or two before bed should be spent with low-key activities, such as taking a bath, watching a low-key TV program, reading, and talking with people who don't stress you out (sorry, mom!).

Talking to Family Members about Your Physical Activity

Playing tennis with a sibling or enjoying a swim with your spouse is a great way to get back into exercising. Other people immediately involve their parents in their exercise routine, or their parents involve themselves. This may be inevitable if you live with your parents. But if they or other family members are overly invested in your mental and physical health, you will find that physical activity becomes aversive. Have a talk with them first to establish guidelines for communicating about exercise. Here are some key points to get across:

• Explain that the best way they can help you is to give you praise for following your new exercise routine but not to be critical or judgmental when you're not. For example, coach your dad not to plead with you or make predictions, such as "You won't be depressed anymore if you go for a swim every day."

• Help them understand that when you're depressed (or coming out of a depressive episode) you need to move at your own pace. They may remember you as a high school athlete, but you're now operating under a much different set of circumstances. Your investment in exercise will probably involve encountering bumps in the road. They need to be flexible in their goals and expectations.

• Make clear what would and wouldn't help in terms of their communication with you. It's fine to say, "I'd like for us to talk about things other than exercise during our calls," or even "Dad, I'd prefer that you not ask me about it." If they insist on progress updates, send them text messages or emails with factual information ("I walked 7,000 steps," "I went to the gym for half an hour").

• For many people, conflict occurs when family members overfocus on their body weight, to the neglect of other aspects of physical and mental health. No one likes to be reminded of being overweight, and the mere mention of it by a parent or spouse can be a trigger for explosive arguments. Explain to them that your weight is a trigger word that inevitably leads to anger. Coach them to talk about your "fitness" rather than "fatness."

• Avoid tying up physical activity with their questions about your medications, doctor appointments, or sleep habits. It's important to keep clear boundaries around discussions of your health habits.

Taking Stock

If you've been able to keep a regular physical activity log, such as the one given earlier, you may start to see the relationship between your activity levels and your mood and sleep. If you have been physically active but are not seeing mood or sleep improvement, it may be time to consider other forms of activity, different frequencies, or different settings.

If you haven't been able to follow through, try not to get down on yourself. It often takes several attempts before regular workout routines become habitual, especially if you haven't exercised for a while. Try to avoid the thinking trap that often comes with physical activity: "I have to wait until I'm not depressed before I exercise." It's easy to think this way because depression makes everything seem heavier. The reality is that exercising will help you come out of the depression if you can "start low and go slow." Exercising with others may create a daily routine that you enjoy, if you're exercising with the right person.

Always keep in mind the ways that your thinking about exercise or physical activity will change when you're stable, depressed, hypomanic, or in between. Your exercise habits may change considerably over time, and there will be starts and stops, forward movement and backsliding. Give yourself plenty of room to mess up; trying to be more active and taking steps in that direction are significant achievements.

11

staying healthy

EATING AND NUTRITION

You're probably familiar with the reasons for maintaining a healthy diet, but BD adds another dimension. People with BD have higher rates of obesity than the healthy population. They are at elevated risk for "metabolic syndrome," usually defined as high blood pressure, excess body fat (particularly around the waist), high levels of blood glucose and insulin, and abnormal cholesterol levels. These are all risk factors for type 2 diabetes, cardiovascular disease, and stroke. Additionally, people with BD who gain weight during treatment have a harder time recovering from mood episodes and more trouble functioning at work or school compared to people with BD who maintain a healthy weight. None of this is good news, but there are things you can do to decrease your risk—other than depriving yourself of your favorite foods.

Prevention Strategies for Moving Toward Healthy Eating

STRATEGY 1: Understand why you have a troubled relationship with food

The first thing you can do is understand why healthy eating is difficult for people with BD. We often read that people with BD have unhealthy lifestyles, drink too much alcohol, use too many drugs, smoke too much tobacco or weed, have erratic

sleep/wake patterns, engage in too little physical activity, and fall prey to their cravings for sugary or overly salty foods. While some of these statements are statisti-
cally true, they don't tell us much about the reasons for this, nor what to do about
them. Worse yet, they make it sound like it's all the person's fault. The literature is
replete with "blame-the-person" statistics. Let's consider some counterarguments:

- The reasons why people with BD have difficulty with food go well beyond
just making the wrong food decisions. When people are cycling into depressive
episodes, they tend to have biologically based cravings for sweets, fried foods, and
lots of carbohydrates and starch. Indeed, intense cravings and poor diets can be
among the warning signs of an oncoming depressive episode. It may be a form of
"self-medicating."

- There are population differences in access to healthy foods. A study of war
veterans found that those with BD were more likely to eat only one meal a day, were
more likely to eat alone, and had more difficulty in obtaining and cooking food than
veterans without psychiatric disorders.

- There are strong genetic predispositions to BD, obesity, diabetes, and cardiovascular disease. That doesn't mean you can't do anything about them, but they
don't occur just because of your food choices. Some of these illnesses are geneti-
cally tied to BD, and many people have obesity, diabetes, or other metabolic disturbances well before their first episode of depression or mania.

- People with BD have to take mood stabilizers, such as lithium or valproate or second-generation antipsychotics (SGAs), such as olanzapine (Zyprexa) or
quetiapine (Seroquel), any of which can increase your appetite and lead to weight
gain. Lithium also causes thirst, which may lead to drinking too many sodas or
other caloric drinks.

STRATEGY 2: Consider medication changes

There are medical strategies to prevent weight gain, regulate glucose, and nor-
malize insulin resistance, all prediabetic signs. Discuss with your doctor whether
you'd benefit from taking Metformin (an antidiabetic agent that normalizes your
response to insulin) in combination with your other medications. If you have gained
a lot of weight on an antipsychotic, talk to your doctor about switching to a less
weight-inducing alternative, such as lumateperone (Caplyta), ziprasidone (Geodon),
aripiprazole (Abilify) or lurasidone (Latuda), keeping in mind that a different antipsychotic may not work as well in controlling your mood swings.

As noted in earlier chapters, medications alone are rarely the only answer to problems that arise in BD. This chapter offers a number of behavioral strategies you can use to eat healthier, while being attuned to the different moods that can lead to over- or undereating or eating the wrong foods. As you'll see, maintaining a healthy weight is not the only reason to keep a good diet: It is also likely to have benefits for your mood, cognitive functioning, energy level, and overall health.

STRATEGY 3: Track your current eating habits

Tracking your diet alongside of your mood, activity, and sleep patterns gives you a lot of information about how your daily and nightly routines are related to each other. You may find that your mood is lower on days in which you eat heavy meals and better when you eat ordinary meals and are more physically active. You can determine whether any of your meals—or what time you ate them—affected your sleep that night or your mood the next day.

Go back to the physical activity and diet chart in Chapter 10 (page 165) and try recording your food and drink intake for the next week (you'll find an example on page 175, the first three lines of which have been filled in). The grid has columns for recording what you ate and drank for breakfast, lunch, dinner, and any snacks you had in between; what your mood was like that day; and your hours of sleep. If you wish, you can add abbreviations to indicate when you "slept poorly" or "did not finish meal." Make a rating of your mood before you had your first meal of the day and after your last one (using the −5 to +5 scale we discussed previously). Recording the time of each meal can be helpful when implementing a time-restricted eating plan (see below).

STRATEGY 4: Construct a healthy eating plan

There are no bipolar-specific diets. Doctors usually recommend "Mediterranean" diets for anyone who is concerned about weight or health: opting for lean protein and good-quality dairy, especially fermented, such as yogurt or kefir, or soft cheese with no added sugars. Eat plenty of fruits, green vegetables, nuts, whole grains, and good-quality protein (like seafood). Most emphasize favoring plant-based foods over processed foods and limiting the amount of saturated fats, trans fats, and salt in your diet. Although the Mediterranean diet is the traditional food of southern Europe and northern Africa, many Asian, Middle Eastern, African, and indigenous American diets have the same features.

If you have (or are at risk for) diabetes, it's best to eliminate sugar from your diet, especially in ultraprocessed foods, such as doughnuts, cakes, and soft drinks, along with processed foods like hot dogs and French fries. Make sure you get

PHYSICAL ACTIVITY AND DIET CHART (EXAMPLE)

Day	Breakfast	Lunch	Dinner	Snacks	Drinks	Physical activity (~ time)	Mood for the day (-5 to +5)	Wake time	Bedtime
Monday	Power bar, banana	Roast beef sandwich	Chicken, green beans, potato	Reese's bar	2 cups coffee, Coke, glass of wine	45 min. walking dog	-1	7:30 am	11:00 pm
Tuesday	Cereal, milk, OJ	Turkey sandwich	Poke bowl	Muffin	2 cups coffee, diet coke, 1 beer	30 min. walking dog	-2	7:15 am	11:30 pm
Wednesday	Cereal, milk, OJ	Salad with chicken	Cheeseburger, fries	Potato chips	2 cups coffee, Sprite, beer	45 min (gym)	+1	7:15 am	11:00 pm
Thursday									
Friday									
Saturday									
Sunday									

enough fiber, which helps regulate glucose uptake by your body and feed microbes that support metabolic health. For more information about healthy diets, stress, and the "mind/gut" axis, I recommend *Food for Thought: Changing How We Feel by Changing How We Eat* by Lisa Goehler (2022).

There is preliminary evidence that ketogenic diets—high in fats, low in carbohydrates, and medium in protein—can help with mood stability in BD. If you want to try the keto diet, work with a dietitian familiar with requirements for brain health to make sure you are getting the daily nutritional requirements. Finally, drink enough water throughout the day, but not so much as to interfere with your lithium levels (8–12 glasses per day is usually recommended). Limit your sugar intake to the equivalent of 6–9 teaspoons per day.

STRATEGY 5: Shop mainly on the outer aisles

Think of your lunch or dinner plate as divided into four equal sections: fruits, vegetables, healthy proteins, and carbohydrates (bread, milk, pasta, potatoes, beans, and juices). Balancing your diet is aided by shopping in the outer aisles of most grocery stores, where you'll find greens, fruits, vegetables, and dairy products.

STRATEGY 6: Avoid fancy diets or eating only one food category

Some people interpret dieting to mean "eat only protein" or "live on nuts and vegetables." You may lose weight in the short term, but almost invariably it'll come back, which can contribute to depression. Also, some diets come with long-term risks, such as an increased risk of heart disease or changes in blood pressure; make sure to read about the long-term as well as short-term effects of any diets you choose.

Strategies for Specific Problems with Eating

? "I feel like my whole evening is centered around eating. After dinner I tend to snack, sometimes equivalent to a whole meal's worth. And then I feel terrible about myself and can't sleep."

PREVENTION STRATEGY 1: Try a time-restricted eating schedule

In Chapter 6, we discussed how people with BD are often phase shifted in their sleep patterns (such as tending to fall asleep after midnight and not being able to wake up before 8:00 A.M.). People with BD tend to be phase shifted in their eating as well, feeling hungry late at night and less hungry early in the morning. Try to shift your eating routines to match the movements of the dark/light cycle. Imagine that you are used to eating your first meal at noon and your last at 10:00 P.M. If you're able to set your body's clock to the light–dark cycle (such as eating your first meal at 7:30 A.M. and your last at 6:00 P.M.), you may see benefits in terms of your moods, weight, and sleep. Start by moving your first meal earlier by half an hour every week (so, in Week 1, eat your first meal at 11:30 A.M. and your last at 9:30 P.M., then move to 11:00 A.M. and 9:00 P.M.). Notice that the number of hours between your first and last meals stays at about 10.

PREVENTION STRATEGY 2: Maximize your noneating hours

Even better, try to aim for 12–14 noneating hours—that is, keep the frame within which you eat anything to about 10 hours, and in which you don't eat to 14. If you have breakfast at 9:00 A.M., dinner at 7:00 P.M., and then don't eat anything from 7:30 P.M. until 9:00 A.M. the next day, you have successfully mastered "time-restricted eating" or "intermittent fasting." This is the same principle as sleep restriction (covered in Chapter 6), in which you sleep for only certain set hours and lie in bed only when you're actually sleeping. Time-restricted eating works only if you truly avoid eating (or drinking anything with calories) in the 12- to 14-hour interval, which is what is hardest. Use your physical activity and diet chart to determine whether time-restricted eating is benefiting your mood, keeping in mind that you may need to do it for a couple of weeks before seeing benefits.

 "My problem is not eating too much; it's that I don't want to eat. Cooking a meal feels like too much work."

In states of depression, people often have no appetite and lose weight fast, sometimes leading to nutritional deficiencies. You may not enjoy food as much when depressed, so you'll be less motivated to prepare foods you like or even to shop for them. You may avoid meals altogether or impulsively order comfort foods from DoorDash, Grubhub, or Uber Eats. These meals come fully prepared from a restaurant and are usually expensive and on the unhealthy side.

PREVENTION STRATEGY 1: Grocery shop once a week on a day that is usually lower in stress for you

If you're depressed to the point of not being able to go to the grocery store, you can usually order healthy foods from the store to be delivered to you.

PREVENTION STRATEGY 2: Try to establish a plan with meals you like that can be put in regular rotation

Keep your meals simple—use recipes with only four or five ingredients that can be cooked in the oven or on the stove without a lot of attention. Stock your freezer with extra servings from dishes that freeze well so you have meals you can just pull out and microwave. Chop lots of veggies for salads and keep them in containers where you can just mix together what you want to eat over a few days.

If you're able to cook but have trouble finding the energy to buy the ingredients, consider delivery companies like HelloFresh or Blue Apron. They mail you a "kit" with fresh ingredients for one to three meals at a time so you don't have to shop for each one.

PREVENTION STRATEGY 3: Eat with others whenever possible

A study in England found that people who regularly ate with others were happier and felt more satisfied with their lives than those who ate alone. Although one could debate whether this is a cause or an effect of one's mood states, social support is one of the strongest protective factors against depression. Of course, doing so requires advance planning. Think creatively about who you could have dinner or lunch with on a regular basis. Trade dinner invites with a couple of steadfast friends or neighbors and, if possible, eat at one another's homes on different nights of the week. If you ordinarily get lunch after a work meeting, ask someone from work to go along with you.

One caveat is that others may encourage you to eat or drink more than you would if you were alone. Some friends always order dessert at restaurants, or another bottle of wine to share that you would just as soon have skipped. If your friend is one such person, you may have to acquaint them with your goals prior to the meal: to consume only a certain number of calories per day, to avoid or minimize alcohol use, or to keep your restaurant bill to a minimum.

IN-THE-MOMENT STRATEGY: Cook while multitasking

If you really don't like to take time for cooking (and many people don't), try to multitask while meal prepping. When you're preparing meals, start by prepping the foods that take the longest to cook, which can include proteins like chicken and fish. While the chicken is in the oven, cut up some vegetables. Some find it easier to cook with a podcast or a book on tape playing in the background.

"When I'm bored or anxious, I start eating and always overeat. Then I feel worse about myself. How do I avoid stress eating when I'm anxious or depressed?"

Depression usually goes along with significant anxiety, and in mixed states (depression with hypomania or mania) anxiety can feel overwhelming. People often impulsively overeat or binge eat to combat anxiety or restlessness. Sometimes the feeling is better described as boredom, which can be hard to distinguish from hunger.

IN-THE-MOMENT STRATEGY: Refocus your attention on a different (and hopefully enjoyable) activity

If you are prone to automatically reach for a snack whenever you feel bored, nervous, or agitated, the simplest in-the-moment strategy is to distract yourself from preparing snacks or simply reaching into a bowl. Storing favorite snacks out of reach, in places far from where you usually store food, will help to interrupt the sequence that leads to automatic eating. If you are having trouble distracting yourself, try an alternative activity: Call a friend, listen to a favorite song, play a video game, or simply spend some time observing your breathing.

PREVENTION STRATEGY 1: Avoid skipping meals, even if you decide to eat less than usual

If you let yourself get too hungry (see Prevention Strategy 2 below), you're more likely to eat out of desperation, which usually means grabbing whatever is easiest. Setting meals at a regular time (see section above on time-restricted eating) makes impulsive eating less likely to occur.

PREVENTION STRATEGY 2: Use mindful eating for appetite awareness

Appetite awareness is a specific strategy to encourage close attention to your physical signals of hunger and fullness before and after you eat. Linda Craighead, professor of psychology at Emory University, developed a program called Appetite Awareness Training for binge or compulsive overeating. The core ideas are to use physical (stomach) signals to guide your eating, such as asking yourself, "Am I really physically hungry, or do I just want to eat for other reasons?" and to stop eating as soon as you feel just full (no longer hungry) instead of eating until you don't *want* anymore. Craighead and her colleagues found that improving appetite awareness leads to less overeating and can give you a greater sense of control over eating.

The program encourages you to make daily ratings of hunger, fullness, and how you feel after you eat. It includes many of the strategies covered in Chapter 1 on depression and cognitive restructuring: flagging instances of negative self-talk; accepting thoughts and behaviors without judgment; and challenging self-talk with alternative, more helpful thoughts.

You may find it most helpful (at least initially) to stop and record your "hunger signals" before and your "fullness" after each time you eat (see the form on pages 181–182). Monitoring your level of hunger and fullness will help you identify instances when you were too hungry and ended up overeating, started eating when you were not really hungry (you saw food or ate for emotional reasons), or ignored your stomach signals and got too full. If you'd like to read more about Appetite Awareness Training, check out *Training Your Inner Pup to Eat Well: Let Your Stomach Be Your Guide,* by Linda Craighead (2017).

Not everything requires filling out a form. You may find it sufficient to track your hunger/fullness mentally through the day and then just rate at the end of the day whether you were able to use stomach signals in guiding your eating. Make a note as to whether there were any eating episodes that didn't feel good physically so you can work on making choices that feel better.

PREVENTION STRATEGY 3: Use mindful eating to experience the food you eat

How can you enjoy eating without becoming obsessive about food, or using eating to manage the difficult emotions that emerge during depressive or manic states? In mindful eating, you use your five senses to fully experience the food you eat. Although it hasn't been shown to bring about weight loss, mindful eating can lead to an enhanced quality of life and well-being and greater satisfaction with your body.

Our work and school lives often require that we eat quickly (or not at all) without much consideration of what we're eating or where it came from. Mindful eating will give you a much different experience of a meal. It involves being in the moment while eating, observing how the meal affects all five of your senses, and expressing gratitude for food and how it was produced. There is nothing religious about this. There are several approaches to mindful eating, but the majority involve the following:

APPETITE AWARENESS TRACKER

1. **Monitoring your appetite:** Notice the physical sensations of hunger and fullness. Distinguish between eating to manage hunger and eating because you just want food. Write down examples of each.

   Helpful examples: You noticed a food craving and waited it out; you stopped eating when you didn't really need any more or weren't enjoying the food.

   Unhelpful: You got too hungry and ended up eating too fast and too much.

2. **Make two ratings each time you eat:**

   Before eating: How hungry or full were you?

Too hungry	Sort of hungry	Not really hungry	Just full	Very full
1	2	3	4	5

   After eating: How hungry or full were you?

Too hungry	Sort of hungry	Not really hungry	Just full	Very full
1	2	3	4	5

3. **At the end of the day:** Rate how much you were able to be mindful and use appetite cues (hunger and fullness) when deciding when, what, and how much to eat.

   Notice food(s) that you wish you hadn't eaten and what might have felt better in that situation.

Not that mindful		Somewhat		Mostly mindful
1	2	3	4	5

   (continued)

4. **Awareness of external stimuli:** Notice the effect of large serving sizes and seeing food and other people eating.

   Helpful example: You used prepackaged servings to limit amounts; you were able to say no to food you didn't really want that much.

   Unhelpful: Others kept eating and you felt you had to do so as well; others ordered dessert or extra alcohol.

5. **Awareness of "What the heck?" responses.**

   Notice and write down unhelpful thoughts like "I don't care," "I'm hopeless," or "I feel rebellious," and then challenge these thoughts.

Unhelpful thoughts	Alternative thoughts
"I've been good all week; I deserve this treat."	"Yes, I've been good all week, and I've been feeling much better physically. I want to stay this way."

6. **Awareness of emotional eating**

   Notice and write down any thoughts or excuses you gave yourself that allowed you to eat for emotional reasons (for example, getting upset by something on social media and eating a lot of ice cream). Describe how you felt after you ate (Was the food worth it? Did you feel better? Or was the food not worth it because you felt worse afterward?).

- Take notice of where the food came from (not only the local grocery store but also who might have grown it, where, and under what conditions). It helps to express gratitude (or imagine expressing it) to those who prepared it, even if they aren't present. It's harder to do this with a frozen dinner, but not impossible.

- Be aware of how the food looks, tastes, and smells, as well as its texture or color. This requires slowing down and taking one bite (or sip) at a time and being attuned to the sensations of the food or drink in your mouth. Of course, this is harder to do if you're in a hypomanic or manic state, but you may also find that doing so helps you slow your mind down.

- Take notice of your setting and how it affects your experience of food. Are others eating quickly, and does that make you want to speed up? If you're alone, do you feel like you need to occupy yourself, such as by checking your phone or reading a book?

- If you are feeling down and are eating alone in a public place, be aware of feeling self-conscious, as if others are wondering why you aren't accompanied. Be aware of these thoughts and don't chase them away, but also ask yourself if they are helpful or unhelpful at that moment.

- If you were hungry when you sat down, notice when you start to feel full, which usually occurs well before you finish what's on your plate. Be aware of the physical sensations of being full. Notice what makes you want to keep eating. If others around you are still eating, you may feel like you should, too.

- If you feel inclined, end the meal with a short gratitude meditation before getting up. An example is *www.youtube.com/watch?v=OCorElLKFQE.*

If you want to learn how to adopt mindful eating practices, I recommend *Savor: Mindful Eating, Mindful Life* by the Zen master Thich Nhat Hanh and Harvard nutritionist Lilian Cheung (2010) or *Eating Mindfully: How to End Mindless Eating and Enjoy a Balanced Relationship with Food* by Susan Albers (2012).

 "How do I stop giving in to cravings?"

IN-THE-MOMENT STRATEGY 1: Choose chewy but low-calorie snacks

If you have any appetite at all during depressive episodes, you may have cravings for high-carbohydrate, high-fat, fried, and processed foods. This is part of the depressive syndrome. You can help avoid excessive snacking by having snack foods that are chewy but low in fat and carbs, such as celery sticks, popcorn, Greek yogurt with berries, olives, pickles, or cottage cheese with pineapple slices. Beef jerky (or plant-based tofu or tempeh jerky) is high in protein but low in fat and carbs and very chewy; these are among the reasons it is easy to find at gas stations when you're on the road. Nuts (almonds, pistachios, and so on) may also satisfy cravings and may even help lower your cholesterol. Be careful of how much salt you eat, however, especially if you're taking lithium. A complete list of snack foods that are nonprocessed, low calorie, flavorful, and high in protein can be found at *www. thehealthy.com/food/stop-the-craving-healthy-snack-ideas*.

You may be surprised that just the act of chewing reduces your anxiety level, even if you aren't satisfying a particular craving. A meta-analysis of eight studies found that chewing gum was associated with decreases in anxiety. Another meta-analysis found that chewing was associated with slight increases in attention and alertness. So chew away!

IN-THE-MOMENT STRATEGY 2: Take it slow

When depressed, it's easy to view the late-night trip to McDonald's as a form of self-reward, but it's one of those rewards that feels good for a few moments and then makes you feel worse. If you have a craving for comfort foods, pause and take a few in-breaths and out-breaths to be fully present with your craving. If you still have cravings after 5 minutes, take about half of the portion of the food you crave from snack foods you have at home (a handful of chips, a scoop of ice cream) and put it on a plate or in a bowl. Eat mindfully, being aware of each bite, leaving time in between bites. The objective here is not to deny yourself all treats, but to apply mindful awareness to all forms of eating, instead of eating impulsively.

 "How do I sort myth from fact about diet in BD?"

Dubious claims abound in the world of dietary advice, and those that pertain to BD are no exception. Here are some prevention strategies to help guide your eating and drinking habits with BD.

PREVENTION STRATEGY 1: Know how to deal with salt and thirst while taking lithium

If you're taking lithium, monitor your salt intake, because any sudden increase or decrease in the amount of sodium you ingest can affect your lithium levels. Avoid low-sodium diets and dehydration, because they can increase your risk of lithium toxicity (a state in which lithium levels go too high, resulting in problems with balance and coordination, mental disorientation, severe diarrhea, stomach pain, blurry vision, slurring of speech, and shaky hands). Talk with your doctor or a nutritionist about how to safely manage the sugar and salt in your diet to stay within a healthy range. Sucking on ice chips and sugarless candy will help with thirst from lithium.

PREVENTION STRATEGY 2: Consume sugar in moderate amounts

There is no evidence that too much sugar causes mania, but there are many health reasons to cut down. First, when you cut down on sugar intake, you will see improvements in your blood pressure, cholesterol, and glucose levels. One way is to cut out added sugars from breakfast, when people often crave sweets. Packaged foods (think premade pancakes) are often loaded with sugar. Try drinking coffee without sugar (or with a sugar substitute) and avoid sugary cereals and soft drinks. Avoid giving in to sugar cravings at the end of the day; if you want dessert, have fruit. If you're used to a lot of sugar and cut down, you may experience craving for the first week or so, but it will lift and you will start feeling more energetic and less irritable.

PREVENTION STRATEGY 3: Have your coffee, but watch the amount

Acute increases in caffeine consumption may precede the occurrence of manic symptoms, either through its stimulating effects, its effects on your sleep patterns, or because of the metabolism of lithium or other medications. Caffeine may suppress lithium concentrations, and, like salt, sudden increases or decreases in your caffeine intake can go along with changes in your lithium levels.

Increases in your coffee intake can actually be a sign of mania or hypomania. When people feel revved up, they are drawn to substances that accentuate the effect. Watch caffeine intake late in the day because it will interfere with your sleep. Aim for one or at most two cups of coffee before noon, and make sure to stop all caffeine after 2:00 P.M.

PREVENTION STRATEGY 4: Don't use omega-3 fatty acids as a mood stabilizer

Omega-3 (fish oil) is not adequate as a mood stabilizer and cannot be substituted for lithium, valproate, lamotrigine, or any of the SGAs. Nonetheless, it can help as an adjunct to your mood stabilizing medications. There is conflicting but mainly positive evidence for the use of omega-3 (and also N-acetylcysteine and inositol) as dietary supplements for bipolar depression. You needn't take omega-3 as a tablet. You can also eat more foods that are rich in omega-3, some of which may not be on your grocery list: walnuts, almonds, wild-caught salmon (or more generally, higher-fat, cold-water fish), sardines, anchovies, spinach, flaxseed, winter squash, and collard greens.

It's important to have a low ratio of omega-6 to omega-3 in your diet. Omega-6 is high in fried foods, along with the vegetable oils they are cooked in. One way to balance omega-6 and omega-3 is to substitute avocado, flaxseed, canola, or olive oil (low in saturated fats) for corn, soybean, safflower, or cottonseed oil when cooking.

Responding to Your Family's Expectations about What You Eat

There are clear risks and benefits of having your family members influence your eating habits. If you are an adult living with one or more parents, chances are that you share at least one meal a day with your parent(s). If you're living with a partner or spouse, it's probably more than one. If you've just come out of the hospital, your living situation may have changed and your access to certain foods may have changed along with it.

A parent or spouse can have a positive influence on your eating habits if they understand the limitations imposed by your disorder, help you plan meals and shopping lists, and have common goals for your (and the family's) health. Those are big *if*s. Having common goals depends on who else shares meals with you, who generally cooks, and who is paying the bills. If you do not agree with your family member(s) on the content or timing of meals, some problem solving may help: Define the problem in a specific way, develop as many solutions as you and they can think of, evaluate the advantages and disadvantages of each solution, home in on one or two solutions, and then make plans to implement the solution(s). The following illustrates how one family of a 21-year-old with bipolar II disorder managed their disagreements on meals:

A Family Problem-Solves Diet Disagreements

Family: Prisha, age 21, is gradually improving after a lengthy episode of bipolar II depression, which forced her to move home during college; sister, Anjali (17), is in high school; mother, Anika, is age 46; and father, Rohan, is 49.

Problem: Prisha wants to become a vegan, partly to advocate for animal rights and partly because she hopes it will help alleviate her depression. Her family eats everything except beef. Prisha wants her mother, who does most of the cooking, to prepare a separate vegan meal for her dinner. Her father doesn't care what Prisha eats but refuses to spend money on two sets of groceries.

Solutions (and who proposed them):

1. Anika cooks a separate vegan meal for Prisha (Prisha)

   Pros: Prisha would get to eat what she wants and the family can eat what they want

   Cons: Mother unwilling to cook a separate meal; the kitchen is not designed to have two meals cooked simultaneously

2. Prisha should move out (Anjali)

   Pros: Anjali and Prisha might get along better, Prisha would like to try living alone

   Cons: Prisha cannot afford to pay rent, and parents are not willing to cover it; parents do not believe she is ready to live independently

3. Prisha should cook for herself (Anika)

   Pros: Mother would not have to cook a separate meal; Prisha would learn more about cooking and taking care of herself

   Cons: Prisha doesn't know how to cook vegan dinners, says she would end up ordering out

4. Prisha should buy and pay for her own groceries (Rohan)

   Pros: Prisha would gain more responsibility; family would not have additional expenses

   Cons: Prisha does not earn enough to pay for all her own meals

5. The whole family should become vegan (Prisha)

   Pros: They would not contribute to animal exploitation in the food industry

   Cons: Everyone else refuses to eat vegan

Solutions chosen: Prisha is to learn how to cook vegan dinners, with Anika's help; in the meantime, Prisha can buy and heat up frozen vegan dinners as long as she pays for them herself. Rohan agrees to contribute funds so that Prisha can buy vegan lunches.

Timeline: Test period of 2 weeks, at which point the family reconvenes and discusses whether solutions have worked. If not, they redefine the problem and start again.

In negotiating meals with your family, be vocal about the limitations imposed by your disorder, which may not affect others in the family. For example, you may have decided to eat more fish as a way of increasing your omega-3 intake. If you live with siblings who hate fish, you may have to prepare your own meals. If you want to try mindful eating, it may be necessary to eat in a different room, especially if others ridicule you for it. Meet your family members halfway where you can, but be assertive about those food choices that are important for your overall health and mood stability.

Taking Stock

By now, you may fear that managing BD means giving up all the foods you like to eat. This is certainly not my intent! All foods are available to you. Few people can make a dramatic transition to a strict diet and stay on it indefinitely. Instead, aim for moderation in your intake of sugar, salt, and caffeine, and make dietary changes gradually, not suddenly. Use a calendar like the physical activity and diet chart in Chapter 10 (page 165) to record your new exercise and eating habits. If you see mood improvement from one change (such as a new exercise program), add other columns as you introduce other changes and expand your definition of improvement to include sleep consistency and feelings of well-being.

Consider how to use these strategies when you're depressed compared to when you're feeling well or hypomanic. If you're like many people, you may have no appetite when depressed, to the point where you are not getting the nutrients you need. Alternatively, depression or anxiety may be associated with overeating, binge eating, or constantly snacking. Try the appetite awareness and mindful eating strategies—even for just a few days—to see how much control you can exert over these behaviors.

Finally, consider not only the food you eat but also the social and familial context in which you eat it. You may have an easier time sticking to a diet if you do it with someone else, or if you divide the shopping chores with your roommate or partner, with instructions not to buy foods that give you trouble. Feeling better about your food consumption and the changes in your body that result will go a long way toward helping you manage difficult mood states.

= 12 =

managing alcohol and substance use

Use of substances—from commonly available things like alcohol and marijuana to harder drugs like cocaine and opioids—is tricky territory for those with BD. The general public is subject to many myths about what's harmful and what's helpful, and there are specific myths about substance use among people with BD. It's important to know why you're choosing to use substances, and how they can affect your health and quality of life (that is, your overall satisfaction or feelings of well-being) with BD. You're probably reading this chapter because you're wondering whether habits that you thought were benign or beneficial really are. Can you live as well as you want to while using substances?

This chapter does not parrot those "Just say no" messages some of us grew up with. Many people occasionally use marijuana, drink, or use drugs, and not everyone suffers ill effects. The reasons people drink or use substances vary: Some say they use them to tamp down difficult emotions, some find that substance use is just a regular part of their social lives, and others just enjoy getting drunk or high. Occasional use of alcohol or drugs is not what is meant by *substance abuse*, which is a more severe habit that occurs daily (or almost daily), interferes with your ability to carry out your ordinary obligations, and gradually dominates your life.

We know that hanging on to substances is one of the things that keeps people with BD from having the quality of life they deserve. The lifetime rate of substance and alcohol use disorders is about 60% in people with BD, compared to 27% in people with major depressive disorder and 17% in the general population. Alcohol and cannabis are used most frequently, followed by cocaine and various opioid pain relievers. This is a major concern, as people with BD who regularly use substances have more mood episodes over time, more suicidality, more rapid cycling, and lower satisfaction with life than those with BD who do not. Consider that your goal of getting your moods stabilized and the competing desire to drink or use drugs might be taking you in opposite directions.

Becoming Aware of What Makes You Use Substances and How Substances Use You

Why do you use substances? Examining your motivations may tell you whether you need to do anything now to control your use or whether the challenges have more to do with risks to your future. This self-awareness can naturally lead to changing your habits or stopping use altogether, to prevent yourself from being "used by substances" or becoming subservient to them. On pages 191–192, you'll find a self-assessment tool for thinking about the things that come before, during, and after your use of your "drug of choice" (DofC). A DofC can be alcohol, marijuana (or CBD oil), a prescription drug (such as Klonopin, Adderall, or oxycodone), or a street drug (like cocaine). Try filling out the tool with reference to the drug that you're most concerned about and refer back to the tool as you read through this chapter.

How to Regulate Your Substance Use to Improve Your Quality of Life

PREVENTION STRATEGY 1: Track your moods and substance use

Despite the warnings about use of substances in BD, many people want to use anyway. Mood episodes can be dismal, and smoking weed or drinking may *temporarily* blunt negative feelings. Try to get a clearer picture of how your use of substances and mood symptoms are related. You can track use of your DofC on your mood chart (much as you did with anger or anxiety) and see how it varies over time with changes in your mood and functioning. When your mood drops, you may start using drugs that elevate it (cocaine is one example), or if you're highly anxious, you may start drinking or using prescription opiates. You may not even realize why you're doing so.

Knowing that mood states are among your triggers for substance use may help with prevention. When your mood is deteriorating and you're craving

SELF-ASSESSMENT TOOL
FOR SUBSTANCE AND ALCOHOL USE

My drug of choice (DofC), may include alcohol:

_____

How often I used it this past week (approximately):

_____

Note: If your DofC is prescribed by your doctor, be realistic as to whether you use it as prescribed or more often than that.

1. What *expectations* drive you toward using your DofC? What do you think you will feel and what will happen? Expectations can range from "I'll feel happier (or less depressed or less anxious)" to "I'll be better able to handle the (work, social, family) situation I'm about to enter" or "I won't be bored."

2. Rate your *level of craving* at any one moment. Use a 1–10 scale where 1 = *I have no desire to use this DofC* and 10 = *I must have it; my craving is uncontrollable.* You may be more comfortable with a simpler scale like 1 = *no desire*, 2 = *some craving*, and 3 = *full* craving (which may include physical sensations of withdrawal).

    To get used to the scale, rate how much craving you feel at this moment: _____

    How much craving did you feel when you woke up this morning? _____

(continued)

3. Make a list of your *triggers* for DofC use. Triggers are those things that make you more likely to use the drug or increase your craving. Triggers may include the presence of certain people with whom you normally drink or get high (and with whom you rarely visit without your DofC); certain places, times of day, or evening; certain routine activities (such as drinking alcohol with meals or smoking weed to help you fall asleep); or using other substances that create the craving (such as alcohol being a trigger for vaping tobacco).

Trigger 1: _____

Trigger 2: _____

Trigger 3: _____

4. Triggers are best managed by *creating* roadblocks—things you do to block your exposure to the trigger. These may include not getting together with certain people with whom you always get drunk or high or figuring out other things to do with them, avoiding alcohol if you're trying to stop smoking, and making your access to the drug more difficult (such as giving it to your partner to store for you).

Roadblock 1: _____

Roadblock 2: _____

Roadblock 3: _____

5. Write down what you would gain or lose by giving up the substance. Losses may include certain friendships or perhaps enjoyment of activities like listening to music. You may also gain things: the money you've been spending on the drug, more interactions with people in which you don't feel impaired, a cleaner driving record.

Gain 1: _____

Gain 2: _____

Gain 3: _____

Loss 1: _____

Loss 2: _____

Loss 3: _____

substances, reaching out to your therapist may help you identify stressors that are operating outside of your awareness (such as relationship conflicts or feelings of rejection). You may want to consult with your psychiatrist to determine whether changes in your medications would help stabilize your moods and, ideally, reduce the potency of mood states as triggers for substance use.

PREVENTION STRATEGY 2: Work on cutting down or cutting out

If your self-assessment indicates that substance use is causing you harm, the most obvious and most simple (and also the hardest) way to prevent harm is to change how much you use. There is no one approach that works for everyone, and different strategies may work better at certain points of your life than at others.

Abstinence—stopping drinking or drug use altogether—is the major tenet of Alcoholics Anonymous (AA) or Narcotics Anonymous (NA) groups for people with "dual diagnoses" (comorbid BD and substance or alcohol use disorders). This approach may be the best option if you've been abusing alcohol or drugs for a long time or your occasional use has morphed into a severe and persistent habit. You may have started using alcohol or substances before your first manic or depressive episode and continued ever since, or you may have developed substance habits after getting discharged from a hospital. Many people with BD swear by AA groups, having found a community of people who understand how difficult it is to remain abstinent. The power of these groups is the social support around remaining sober and the community pride in doing so.

Nonetheless, AA or NA groups are not for everyone, and it's important to find the right group for your needs (assuming you have a choice). Some find it hard to be with people who are confirmed alcoholics or drug users. One patient of mine put it this way: "I can't go to groups where people talk about all the glorious things they did when they were high. It just makes me want to use more." You may feel more comfortable in groups of people who are close to your age and level of functioning. Additionally, avoid groups that give the message that dependence on any drug, psychiatric or not, is an addiction. We know this not to be true—people do not become addicted to mood stabilizers or antipsychotics. If you attend meetings where this message is presented as fact, find another meeting.

Another approach is called *harm reduction*, which involves modulating use rather than aiming to stop. You implement strategies to reduce your craving (prevention) and put up roadblocks to manage triggers in the moment. My aim is aligned with this view: to help you reduce the frequency and impact of your use so that your overall health doesn't deteriorate. I believe this strategy has been more effective and realistic for the majority of people with BD that I've worked with, especially those who have had only a few mood episodes and for whom substance use is not yet a long-standing problem.

PREVENTION STRATEGY 3: Know the facts about the relationship between BD and substance use

There are many myths about BD and substance use or abuse, and it's important to know what has and hasn't been established in research studies. Here are a few of those myths:

- "Drinking or taking drugs is about self-medicating." Many people with BD say they use alcohol or drugs to manage their mood symptoms—what we call *self-medicating*. While this explanation might seem logical, it isn't supported by the evidence, which consistently shows that alcohol and drugs make mood episodes worse in BD, not better. Using substances leads to longer and more frequent mood episodes, increased suicidal behavior, more inconsistent use of psychiatric medications, and a lower overall quality of life.

- "Alcohol and drugs can bring you down from a manic episode." If anything, the opposite is true: People use cocaine or marijuana to accentuate the manic state. There is also evidence that alcoholism can precipitate manic episodes in some people.

- "Marijuana is a good mood stabilizer." Many people believe that substances like cannabis are good mood stabilizers and work as well as lithium. This is not the case. People report feeling temporarily better after smoking marijuana (for some, less anxious), but there is substantial evidence that chronic cannabis use is associated with a poorer outcome of BD, with worsening of depression, mania, psychosis, and suicidality. The negative effects are more pronounced when people use cannabis instead of mood stabilizers or antipsychotics.

- "Substance abuse and bipolar disorder are the same illness." It is certainly true that the two co-occur often, and often run in the same families, but many disorders are comorbid with BD, including anxiety disorders and attention-deficit/hyperactivity disorder (ADHD). Substance abuse disorders and BD follow different courses over time and have different ages of onset. In some people, the substance or alcohol abuse predates the onset of BD, and in others the BD comes first.

PREVENTION STRATEGY 4: Aim for greater mood stability

"I don't like spending money on drugs or booze, but my mood-stabilizing medications just don't seem to help enough."

If you find that your use of your DofC increases when you're depressed or (hypo) manic—or in the prodromal phases of either state—you are probably also facing financial distress related to substance use. If so, getting stable from your existing mood symptoms should be your first priority, for both financial and physical health reasons. Talk to your doctor about why your existing medications are not doing what they should. Your medication regimen may not be optimal, and your doctor may recommend dosage changes or additions. As always, seek a second opinion if your doctor has run out of ideas. Your doctor may be right that your drug or alcohol use is interfering with the potential benefits of your medications, but you may have originally turned to substances because you weren't experiencing any medication benefits.

Consider a monthlong experiment where you give up (or greatly reduce) your use of your DofC to see how your mood changes. If you have doubts about whether you can do this, consider more aggressive treatments (as recommended by your doctor) that you've avoided up until now, such as antipsychotics (which have been shown to reduce cravings) or Antabuse (which makes you sick when you drink alcohol). Many people are surprised to learn that they have some control over their cravings and whether they act to satisfy them.

What You Can Do about Cannabis Use

 "Weed is harmless and helps with my anxiety, so why should I stop using it?"

I often hear statements like this, or the related idea, "I'd rather keep using weed instead of mood stabilizers since it does the same thing and it's available over the counter, so it must be safer." The legalization of marijuana in many states has supported people's beliefs that there is nothing dangerous about the drug—as mentioned above, many people with BD use it every day and substitute it for mood stabilizers or antipsychotics.

PREVENTION STRATEGY: Know the facts about cannabis

Here are some facts about cannabis that should inform your decision to use or not use it regularly:

1. **Safety.** Smoking, vaping, or eating marijuana on occasion is not particularly dangerous for a person with BD, but there are a number of caveats. The high-potency THC (delta-9-tetrahydrocannabinol, one of the main active ingredients in marijuana) available on the street and in dispensaries is associated with a higher risk of psychotic symptoms, anxiety, and depression. Some of the cannabis products available today—including cannabidiol (CBD) gummies—have THC in them, even if it may not say so on the package. It's important to know exactly what you're buying.

2. **Effects on mood and anxiety.** Marijuana may have pleasant, short-term calming effects on your anxiety, but with repeated and chronic use it can depress your mood, contribute to feeling low in energy and motivation, and increase your anxiety. THC has been shown over and over to impair memory, attention, verbal learning, and processing speed (the time taken to respond to visual or verbal information).

3. CBD, the other major ingredient in marijuana, is usually marketed as CBD oil. It has different effects on the brain from THC and appears more likely to reduce anxiety, but we know little about its long-term effects. The coexistence of these two compounds is one of the reasons that marijuana has such unpredictable effects.

4. **Regular use of cannabis** can interfere with your psychiatric medications and contribute to making your moods and cognition worse. If you are looking to cannabis to help you chill out, consider mindful meditation practices for your anxiety states, as described in Chapter 3.

5. **Influence of others.** Use of cannabis has a strong environmental component. If your social life revolves around cannabis use (that is, most of your friends smoke weed), you may find that you crave cannabis more when with them than when alone. What relationships or activities might you be giving up if you stopped smoking? These influences are especially strong when others around you use weed to calm themselves in social situations.

6. **Motivation and personal goals.** Consider how your use of weed affects achievement of your personal academic, health, or work goals. If you use it daily, you may recognize that you don't achieve certain objectives you had at the beginning of the day (such as to exercise or finish a work assignment) because of cannabis use. If you use it regularly during the work week, you may observe a gradual decrease in your work motivation or productivity. Reducing your use—like using it only with friends on weekends—may produce a corresponding increase in motivation and goal directedness during the week.

7. **What happens to your anxiety when you don't smoke?** If you are a regular cannabis user (vaping or eating some almost every day), try an experiment like the one described in Prevention Strategy 4 (above). Rate your daily level of anxiety on your mood chart for 1 week while using cannabis as you regularly do (and sticking with your psychiatric medications as prescribed). Then try 1 week without weed and make the same ratings. Although you may experience anxiety at first, you may be surprised that it isn't as hard as you thought. If you can't stop by choice, talk to your doctor about whether you're a candidate for the antianxiety agent gabapentin, which is nonaddictive and can treat anxiety related to cannabis use.

 "When I'm feeling hypomanic, I smoke weed to feel calmer. Why does that seem to backfire?"

PREVENTION STRATEGY: Take protective measures, especially during hypomania or mania

It's tempting to believe that, because cannabis can have a short-term calming effect, it must also be antimanic. When you smoke weed (or use any other drug, for that matter), prepare for any way it can go wrong and be honest with yourself about your limits. You may be more prone to impulsive decision making and risk taking when high. If your moods are not being stabilized with agents like lithium or valproate, you may use weed in more dangerous situations. It can also disturb your sleep and lead to the impulsive behaviors that are a run-up to mania (like having sexual encounters without caution or spending money impulsively).

If you're currently hypomanic and determined to keep using cannabis, try taking a trip to a legal dispensary (if available in your area). The cannabis products you buy in regulated dispensaries are likely to be cleaner than those you buy on the street. If the dispensary has helpful individuals working the counter, ask them about types of cannabis that don't contribute to feeling wound up. You needn't explain your disorder; you can simply say "I sometimes get lots of energy—can you recommend a type of weed that isn't activating?"

Harm Reduction for Alcohol Use

Like marijuana, the occasional drink is not going to hurt you. Most psychiatrists will tell you that a glass of wine with dinner is OK. But what about when occasional use turns into abuse? How can you reduce the number of heavy drinking episodes?

Alcohol abuse and BD are a toxic combination. Alcohol certainly worsens mood swings and interacts negatively with medications, such as lithium. People with BD who abuse alcohol and harder drugs like cocaine are more likely to die prematurely than people with BD who don't use substances, for reasons that include overdosing (accidental and purposeful), accidents, and declining health.

Whereas the goal in 12-step groups like AA is to remain sober at all times and never drink again, a typical harm reduction goal is to reduce your frequency of heavy drinking episodes (usually defined as five or more drinks in a single night) to zero, even if you continue to have evenings of lighter drinking. People with BD who are at highest risk for impairment from alcohol are often light drinkers who go through periods of heavy drinking, such as during depressive episodes. But reducing heavy drinking episodes requires thinking about the context.

PREVENTION STRATEGY 1: Manage relationships with the people who make you want to drink

We all need a community and a sense of support from others, but if your social life revolves around drinking, the obvious strategy is to avoid the people or places where drinking is more likely to occur. That may mean giving up certain drinking buddies or developing camaraderie with them around some other activity. This is not easy and can be a hurdle. Here are some questions to consider:

- What are the ways that your current social life has supported your goal of living well with BD? Can you find a community that supports your desire to reduce drinking or stop altogether? I am not suggesting you go out and join a church, but there may already be people in your social network who would be happy to spend time with you without having to drink.

- What are some ways you can enjoy being with your usual friends without drinking? You may be able to think of things you could do that don't involve alcohol (or another DofC). Of course your friend may sabotage the activity by showing up drunk or high. Can you imagine being with that person without one or both of you being high? If not, what does that tell you about the relationship?

- A particularly challenging experience is being in a romantic relationship with someone who requires drinking to enjoy themselves. If you're in such a relationship or developing one, you may want to test it by determining whether the other person wants to see you in settings where drinking is difficult or impossible (such as going hiking or biking). If they decline, it's time for a conversation.

PREVENTION STRATEGY 2: Take the medical approach to alcohol

If your substance or alcohol use is severe and you're having trouble controlling it, and especially if it's destabilizing your moods, talk to your psychiatrist about whether you are a candidate for drugs used to treat alcohol addiction. As mentioned above, Antabuse (disulfiram) is a deterrent to alcohol use because it makes you sick when you drink. Two other agents—naltrexone (Vivitrol or Revia) and acamprosate (Campral)—have been found to reduce relapses into drinking in people with alcohol abuse. Naltrexone blocks the euphoric effects of alcohol, reduces cravings, and gradually reduces the desire to drink; acamprosate reduces anxiety during withdrawal. These agents can be quite effective but also have side effects. They should be combined with alcohol counseling programs to be maximally effective.

In-the-Moment Damage Control

Along with longer-term prevention strategies, there are things you can do in the moment to reduce the damage done to yourself or others from drinking alcohol or using substances. These strategies are harder to implement when you're heading into mania or hypomania, but enumerating them when you're stable will help you bring them to mind when you're symptomatic, much as you did when restructuring daily routines or sleep habits.

STRATEGY 1: Put up roadblocks

If friends have invited you to a party or a concert on a Saturday night and you know you're likely to drink, consider limiting yourself to one beer. Some people like the taste of nonalcoholic beer, which is another option. Alternatively, simply decline to drink or explain that you're trying to lose weight or have to get up early the next day. Depending on the nature of your friendships, this may be all the explanation required.

STRATEGY 2: Avoid testing your ability to manage small amounts of your DofC

Understandably, people often believe that substance use is safe when their moods are stable, but challenge yourself when thinking, "How about I try a little of my drug of choice since I'm feeling OK?" As you probably know from prior experience, it doesn't work that way. Regular use of alcohol, cocaine, opiates, or other drugs of abuse can lead to the alteration of reward pathways in the brain that regulate dopamine, even when you're feeling fine. These alterations can put you at greater risk for relapses of both substance abuse and mania.

STRATEGY 3: Contact a source of emergency help

If you're prone to using your DofC while alone, and especially if you're feeling suicidal when doing so, use emergency phone numbers or mobile apps to keep yourself safe. Never Use Alone (*www.neverusealone.com*; 877-696-1996) consists of volunteers who have experience with substance abuse themselves. When you call, they will stay on the phone with you while you're using and for about 10 minutes afterward to make sure you're OK. If you stop responding and they can't reach you, they will call the emergency medical services in your area.

You can also contact The Brave App (*www.thebraveapp.com*), which can help prevent a drug overdose. When you contact them (through a button on the app) for the first time, you set up a rescue plan with details such as where you live and who should respond in an emergency. If you are in the midst of a drug experience and become unresponsive by phone, they will call your designated family member or friend or send an emergency medical person (as written in your rescue plan). They will try to honor your request not to involve the police, but they may not have control over who shows up with an ambulance.

Communicating with Family Members

 "All they want to talk to me about is my drinking."

As with all things bipolar related, family members play a significant role in alcohol and substance use problems. The key with family members is to make sure they know to balance their communication with you so that they aren't constantly hounding you about taking your meds, going to AA meetings, or seeing your doctor. The hounding can itself be a trigger for your cravings and substance use.

PREVENTION STRATEGY 1: Regulate communication with family

PREVENTION STRATEGY 1A: If your parent or partner wants to talk to you about your drug or alcohol use, set a time during the week where you talk about that and only that

You might say, "During Sunday dinner you can ask me things like 'Did you take your meds and have you seen your doctor or gone to an AA meeting?' Other times we talk about other things."

PREVENTION STRATEGY 1B: If you've had repeated recurrences of substance or alcohol abuse and are now sober, you may need to reorient your parent(s) to where you are in development so that they communicate with you as an adult

That also means avoiding responding as you might have when you were a teenager (such as by using alcohol or drugs to get revenge, or cursing when they bring the topic up). Note that you'll be on shakier ground here if you're repeatedly relapsing into drug or alcohol abuse and your parents or other family members have had to intervene in dangerous situations.

PREVENTION STRATEGY 1C: Communicate clearly with a spouse or partner

Say, "It's not your job to fix me. You can drive me to appointments or to the drugstore, but it's me who has to go in and see my doctor or fill my prescriptions. You can't do this for me." Likewise, your partner shouldn't be tracking your drinks or running urine tests on you, which turns them into your doctor (or jailer) rather than your partner.

PREVENTION STRATEGY 1D: Try to reorient your partner to the relationship you had when you first got together

What did you enjoy doing together? You can say, "Let's have conversations like we used to. I'm a person independent of my illness. I'm not just an alcoholic; I'm a person with bipolar disorder and alcoholism, and I'm also a _____ [husband, teacher, musician, father, or however else you describe yourself]."

PREVENTION STRATEGY 1E: Make sure your spouse or family members are not using alcohol or drugs in your presence

If your family can only spend time together while drinking, this may not be a viable situation for you if you're trying to cut down. Spend time with them in the morning, when people are less likely to get high or drink.

PREVENTION STRATEGY 1F: Be clear that the questions posed by your spouse/partner or family members are probably coming from a place of fear

When they ask, out of the blue and with no evidence, "Have you been drinking today?" you can respond accordingly: "I know you're worried about my drinking, and your fears are understandable. But I'd rather talk about my problems with alcohol in my next AA group (or with my therapist/alcohol or drug counselor)."

The points to make clear:

- I am a person—I'm your son/daughter (brother/sister/husband and so on).
- I don't want to be treated as just an illness or a brain disease.
- If I have an ordinary mood change, don't immediately ask me if I'm drunk or high or if I've missed my meds.
- I have normal fluctuations in my moods that are due to stress, just like everyone else.

Taking Stock

If you've had an opportunity to track your triggers and cravings on your mood chart or on the self-assessment tool (pages 191–192), look at the past week and determine what went well and what didn't. Are there situations or feelings (triggers) that you're trying to avoid that lead to craving and use? Certain people with whom you always get high? Predictable periods of time or places where craving hits its peak? Were your expectations for using the substance fulfilled? Did any of the roadblocks work for decreasing your use? Use this information in the next week to avoid those triggers and reduce periods of craving.

As you're going through the process of managing triggers and cravings, there are bound to be slipups, and hopefully those will become less frequent over time. So, try to keep the "30,000-foot view" in mind: Ask yourself whether your current pattern of alcohol or substance use is helping you get what you want (the job, the relationship, greater stability) and in what ways it's interfering. Regulating substance abuse involves being continuously conscious of what you want for yourself in the long term, even when other desires present themselves in the moment.

PART THREE

your treatments

MAKING THE MOST OF MEDICATIONS AND THERAPY

When you read about treatment recommendations for BD on the internet or in books, you may feel like the information is well-intentioned but dismissive. Not every problem needs to be treated with a pill or with psychotherapy. Some of what you're coping with is just part of the human condition, and some mood changes come about because of stress in your environment. Availing yourself of treatment options doesn't mean you're admitting that this is all your fault or all in your head. As you'll see, you have more agency than you might think in developing a treatment plan. In this part, you'll learn some strategies for establishing a proper medication regimen, advocating for yourself in modifying it, and making psychotherapy work for you.

13

taking charge of your medications

Most, if not all, people with BD have struggled with taking medications—whether to take them at all and, if so, whether they work or not, how to cope with side effects, their effects on physical health, and the inevitable stigma of taking them. I don't think I've worked with anyone who got the right medication on the first try and stuck with it.

Mood-stabilizing medications are a boon to those living with BD. In earlier eras, before lithium came on the scene, people with BD were in and out of hospitals. Lithium allowed people to be treated on an outpatient basis and enjoy a much more satisfying life. Nowadays there are many more options than lithium, but getting the right regimen takes time and often means a lot of trial and error and seeing more than one specialist. Even then, meds can't resolve every problem that you're living with.

It can be hard to commit to taking medications if you don't believe they're effective, you have intolerable side effects, or those close to you attribute all or most of your problems to inadequate medications. People with BD often have very stressful lives. If you frequently hear that your life would be easier if you were just on the right medications or on higher dosages, or if you took them more consistently, you will probably want to dump the medications and start all over. You may wonder whether the treatment is worse than the disease. Here are some statements I have heard from my patients who have struggled with medications:

"I'm expected to be this passive pill swallower, not ask questions, and just go along with the program. I've never been passive about anything; why would I be about something this important?"

"The drugs even out my highs and lows, but am I supposed to just accept the side effects? Are the benefits worth the costs?"

"After all this trial and error, will I ever find the right combination and get the benefits I want?"

"Everyone, from my doctors to my family members, has a say in what drugs I take, when and how much, except for me."

There are volumes of studies that show that, if you're on an optimal set of medications, you'll have fewer mood episodes and fewer symptoms between episodes (see Goldberg and colleagues, 2022, for a recent review). The same is true of added psychotherapy, as long as it's aimed at helping you understand the disorder, adopt relevant lifestyle strategies, and cope with stress triggers in your daily life. But neither is a cure-all. Even optimal medications can leave gaps in symptom management, cause difficult side effects, or make you feel like you can't fully access your emotions or your natural creativity. Medications and therapy are *tools*, options you can avail yourself of—but you're the one who should be in charge. That's why I've labeled the recommendations in this chapter and the next as "taking control" strategies.

Practical Strategies for Taking Control of Your Treatment

 "Ever since I was first diagnosed, everyone has told me I have to take medications. But I'm still not convinced. How do I figure out which ones to take or whether to take them at all?"

Many people with a bipolar diagnosis take time to agree to a medication regimen. Your first experiences with medications may have been in the hospital, where you didn't have much choice. Possibly, you were much younger when your parents first insisted that you take a mood stabilizer or antidepressant. As an adult, it makes sense to make a well-informed decision about whether to take medications and which ones to take—in other words, to take control of your own treatment.

Ideally, you can rely on your doctor to help weigh the costs and benefits of this decision. Unfortunately, in today's medical environment many doctors don't have much time to spend with patients, and you might leave an appointment feeling like you have more questions than answers. Additionally, it is difficult to agree to a medication plan while also being uncertain about whether you have bipolar illness. If the diagnosis is new to you and you have doubts about whether it applies to you, seek a second opinion from another provider, especially if you feel that the first diagnosis was done hastily. But as you'll soon see, deciding whether to take medications goes well beyond whether you meet the rather complicated diagnostic criteria of the *Diagnostic and Statistical Manual of Mental Disorders, Fifth Edition, Text Revision* (DSM-5-TR; 2022).

The following strategies will help you obtain reliable information about medical treatments for BD and clarify your position on taking medications, independent of what others think.

TAKING CONTROL STRATEGY 1: Review your past experiences with mood episodes

Taking medications is much easier when you feel like the choice has been yours based on a reasoned evaluation of your history with mood swings, rather than feeling burdened by the wishes, beliefs, or demands of others. Revisit the chapter on mood charting (Introduction) as well as Chapters 1 and 2 to review the effects that mood changes have had on your relationships, career goals, sleep, and other aspects of daily life. If you've been on mood-stabilizing medications before, you may have opinions on whether they've been effective in stabilizing your prior episodes or reducing recurrences.

TAKING CONTROL STRATEGY 2: Gather as much information as you can

Taking versus not taking medications may feel like less of a choice than what medications you take and at what dosage, weighing the side effects with the potential benefits. Through your own research (from reputable websites or other informed sources) and through discussions with your doctor, you'll be in a better position to clarify your beliefs about which medications to take, at what dosages, and for what purposes.

The tables on page 208 offer basic information on medications used for BD during manic or depressive episodes. There are other sources that provide more detail (for example, see *www.dbsalliance.org/pdfs/medication_charts/BPmedication_chart.pdf*). It's unlikely that you'll end up trying all of these drugs, but you may be on some of them, alone or in combination. Your regimen can also change over time.

It's helpful to know what symptoms each drug targets. For example, you

Medications for Manic Episodes of Bipolar Disorder

Generic name	Brand name (examples)	Starting dosages	Full daily dose
Lithium	Eskalith-CR	600–900 mg	900–2,400 mg
Valproate	Depakote, Depakote-ER	750 mg	1,000–3,000 mg
Risperidone	Risperdal	2 mg	4–6 mg
Quetiapine	Seroquel	100–200 mg	300–800 mg
Olanzapine	Zyprexa	5–10 mg	10–30 mg
Ziprasidone	Geodon	40–80 mg	120–160 mg
Aripiprazole	Abilify	5–10 mg	10–30 mg
Asenapine	Saphris	10 mg	10–20 mg
Carbamazepine	Equetro	200–400 mg	600–1,600 mg
Haloperidol	Haldol	2–5 mg	5–20 mg

Note. Not listed are various classes of antidepressant medications that are used as adjunctive agents. From *Clinician's Guide to Bipolar Disorder* (p. 69) by D. J. Miklowitz and M. J. Gitlin. Copyright © 2014 The Guilford Press. Adapted by permission.

Medications for Depressive Episodes of Bipolar Disorder

Generic name	Brand name (examples)	Starting dosage	Full daily dose
Quetiapine	Seroquel	50–100 mg	200–600 mg
Lurasidone	Latuda	20–40 mg	20–120 mg
Lamotrigine	Lamictal	25 mg	100–400 mg
Lithium	Eskalith-CR	300–600 mg	900–1,800 mg
Valproate	Depakote	250–500 mg	1,000–2,000 mg
Olanzapine/fluoxetine combination	Symbyax	6–25 mg	6/25–12/50 mg
Olanzapine	Zyprexa	5 mg	5–15 mg
Lumateperone	Caplyta	42 mg	42 mg
Cariprazine	Vraylar	1.5 mg	1.5–3.0 mg

Note. Not listed are various classes of antidepressant medications that are used as adjunctive agents. From *Clinician's Guide to Bipolar Disorder* (p. 90) by D. J. Miklowitz and M. J. Gitlin. Copyright © 2014 The Guilford Press. Adapted by permission.

might be prescribed lamotrigine for depression or anxiety, but it is unlikely to be the first choice for hypomania or mania since lamotrigine has no known efficacy to treat or prevent those illness phases. For the latter, doctors usually recommend lithium, valproate, or one of the antipsychotics.

"How do I get information from my doctor about what my meds are doing, whether they're working, and what side effects to expect?"

TAKING CONTROL STRATEGY 1: Be direct about your desire for information

No doctor should just throw medications at you without an explanation of why these drugs are being recommended; what symptoms they treat (mood, sleep, agitation, and so on); what side effects are most likely to occur at these dosages; and whether any other medication, psychotherapy, or device-based option (like transcranial magnetic stimulation [TMS]) should be considered. You should bring up other medications you're taking to find out if there are any drug interactions (for example, birth control pills can make lamotrigine less effective by speeding its metabolism).

If you have a regular psychiatrist (recommended) or other prescriber, these are topics to have an ongoing discussion about, not just once. You can diplomatically pose questions like those in the box at the bottom of the page. Avoid asking them in an accusatory way because, like all human beings, your doctor may get defensive. Medication management sessions are usually shorter than therapy appointments, but ask your questions anyway.

Beware of physicians who "mansplain," which, despite the terminology, can emanate from doctors of either sex: detailed and condescending explanations for things you already know (for example, what bipolar means, what mania is; see the example in the box on pages 211–213). If you feel your doctor is talking down to you

---

Questions to Address with Your Doctor Concerning Medications

- What symptoms are the prescribed medications treating? For example, do they treat sleep problems as well as moods? Energy level as well as emotions?

- How will we know if these are the right ones? What other agents (or treatment methods) are we considering?

- How long before we'll know which drugs are working?

- Which side effects can I expect at these dosages? Which ones will occur mainly at the beginning and which ones will persist?

- What are the best strategies for dealing with bothersome side effects?

- Do any of the medications being prescribed interact negatively with other medications I'm taking?

or telling you things you already know, redirect them by asking direct and specific questions: Why lithium, or why an antipsychotic? How do you cope with difficult side effects? If you're taking more than one agent, how will you and your doctor decide that one agent isn't adding to the other?

In the example, the doctor is initially terse and reticent, but gradually warms up and rewards Kendra's persistence. Not all doctors require prodding but some do. If you feel uncomfortable about having had to exert effort to get critical information from your doctor, or they seem harried or impatient and you are not getting your questions answered, tell them how important it is to feel like a partner in your own treatment. What is their approach to addressing questions about your medications?

If you're consistently frustrated by their answers or feel that they're blowing you off, find a different provider. Sadly, the majority of people with BD consult an average of four different providers before getting a proper diagnosis, let alone an effective treatment.

TAKING CONTROL STRATEGY 2: Check out online drug information and make a list of questions

Although your doctor should provide enough information to go on, you can also find voluminous information online about each drug, what they're supposed to be doing, and what side effects to expect. There are also chat rooms and email list-servs in which you can correspond with others who have taken these meds. Chat groups are available through the Depression and Bipolar Support Alliance (*www.dbsalliance.org*), WebMD (*www.webmd.com*), National Alliance on Mental Illness (*www.nami.org*), and the International Bipolar Foundation (*https://ibpf.org/social-media-communities*).

Obtaining information through websites or social media chat groups also has risks. Be especially skeptical of online postings that aren't vetted for accuracy, which often appear on popular sites such as Reddit or TikTok. There are online forums that push unreliable information or spread unfounded conspiracy theories about predatory drug companies, profiteering doctors, or medications that presumably destroy your brain cells. Someone who posts a negative treatment experience online may have had circumstances that don't necessarily translate to other people, or they may form questionable conclusions about what they think went wrong in their treatment. The other side can be apparent as well: sites that are managed by the drug company that makes a certain medication may play down side effects or play up effectiveness. So, know the sources you obtain information from, look for consistency in recommendations across different sites, and avoid making major health care decisions based on anything you read from random postings.

How to Communicate with Your Provider: An Example

Scenario: It's the first outpatient session for Kendra, age 27, who is recovering from a manic episode with mixed (depressive as well as manic) features. She was initially seen by her general practitioner, who, after a failed trial of clonazepam (Klonopin), recommended she see a specialist in BD. Her new psychiatrist has reviewed her moods and family history. He suggests lithium, a common enough recommendation but one that raises a lot of questions for Kendra, who has never taken it before. She comes in with a basic knowledge of mood-stabilizing medications. In this exchange she makes it clear that she expects to have a participatory role in her own treatment and especially that she wants clarity on what to expect as she adjusts to the regimen. She is persistent but not abrupt or accusatory.

DOCTOR: I'm writing you a prescription for lithium. I'm starting you on 600 mg, and we'll go up by 300 every week or so to a target dose of 1,200 mg, which is four tablets a day. We should meet every 2 weeks while you're getting adjusted, and you'll need to get a lithium level drawn at a lab before our next meeting. How does that sound? (*Closes note-taking book*)

KENDRA: Thank you. Can you tell me more about lithium and why you're recommending it?

DOC: Well, as I mentioned, I think you have bipolar I disorder. That's a disorder where people's moods go up and down in extremes. . . .

KENDRA: (*Politely interrupting*) Yes, that part I understand. What I'd like to know is why you're recommending lithium.

DOC: (*Pauses*) Well, lithium is the oldest medication we have and one of the most effective and best tolerated for bipolar disorder. It's meant to even out the highs and lows but is particularly helpful for stabilizing the highs. And since you're coming off of a high with some elevation of mood, I think that's the best choice.

KENDRA: OK, that's helpful. But why lithium over alternatives like Lamictal or Depakote?

DOC: I can see you already know some things about these medicines. Let me explain a little further. While all of these medicines are informally called "mood stabilizers," that name is something of a misnomer because they all do different things. Lamictal has no known value to treat or prevent mania—it's more useful against depression. Depakote is a good option for treating mania in the active phase, but it's less certain that it can prevent new manic episodes like lithium can. I can refer you to a good website if you want to learn more. (*Stands up*)

KENDRA: (*Persisting*) OK, I realize I'm asking a lot of questions, but once I understand the treatment plan it'll be easier for me to stick with it. For example, why lithium and not one of these newer drugs I see advertised on TV, like Caplyta or Vraylar?

DOC: (*Sits down again*) Some experts believe that if lithium is going to work, its best chance is in the first few episodes, so I prefer to see it tried sooner rather than later. Lithium works extremely well in reducing symptoms, and may also reduce your risk of future episodes. We can consider drugs like Caplyta or Vraylar later if you're not getting the effects we want from lithium, and especially if you have depressive symptoms that won't lift. But those medicines have side effects that can be tough for some people.

KENDRA: OK, I'll have more questions about that, but can you tell me more about the side effects of lithium?

DOC: Everything, unfortunately, has the possibility of causing side effects—even placebos can do that. Because lithium is a salt, you might find your mouth gets dry and you're thirstier, so you may drink more, and if you drink more, you'll have to urinate more often. Let me know if that happens, because there are ways to manage that problem if it comes up. Another possible side effect is hand tremor (demonstrates). If that happens, we might lower the dose or add another medicine to counteract it.

KENDRA: (*Nodding*) What else?

DOC: Don't skimp on your intake of table salt, because if that happens, your body may retain too much lithium and the level could get higher than we want it to. If your level becomes too high, you would also have gastrointestinal side effects like nausea, stomach cramps, or diarrhea.

KENDRA: Oh boy, I can't wait! This isn't sounding like such a wonderful drug to me.

DOC: (*Smiles*) I understand your reaction. I'm letting you know about possible side effects that are of concern, and I'm not suggesting you'll develop all of them. We'll watch for these things early on to make sure the drug is safe for you as you acclimate to it.

KENDRA: OK, I've also heard about "blunting of emotions" with lithium, that it can make you tired or like, flattened out.

DOC: I'm glad you mentioned that because it may be part of lithium's urban legend more than anything else. So long as blood levels don't become too high, cognitive side effects like feeling dull with lithium are rare. In fact, lithium is known to protect nerve cells in the brain from damage and may even have some benefits on attention and memory. We certainly are not aiming to cause blunted emotions, so if you start to feel this is happening, let me know and we'll discuss it.

KENDRA: Well, I play the violin, and music is very important to me. I'd like to avoid anything that might make me feel less creative or slowed down. Also, the shaking of the hands concerns me.

DOC: (*Pauses*) I didn't know you were a musician. You know, studies have shown that people who have bipolar disorder often score high on measures of creativity and tend to have a presence in the art world. If anything, we'd hope that better management of your moods would allow your creative self to flourish.

KENDRA: Thank you. What about weight gain?

DOC: Lithium can sometimes cause weight gain. If it happens, it's usually a slow, gradual process, so when I see you for follow-up appointments we'll weigh you, and I'll be asking about your diet and physical activity. If your weight does start to creep up, we can add antidote medicines to counteract weight gain. And, of course, if we think lithium isn't helping, we'll move on to something else altogether.

KENDRA: OK, one more. I realize it's hard to predict, but what is your strategy for deciding when to stop a drug like lithium and substitute something else? How will I know if it's working?

DOC: It's a good question. I don't follow one strategy; it really depends on the individual, how quickly they get to therapeutic blood levels, and whether their moods are getting stable or not. I like to give it at least a month or two.

KENDRA: Thanks. I'm sure next time I'll have dozens more questions, but I like to be clear on what I'm agreeing to healthwise.

DOC: Understood. Might I suggest that you keep a log of any concerns that might come up between now and the next time I see you so we can make sure we've covered everything?

This is one of many discussions that Kendra will have with her doctor. She has communicated that she is an informed consumer and wants to minimize the effects of lithium on her day-to-day life.

Your online fact finding should suggest questions to ask your doctor at the next appointment. You may be able to send a list of such questions to your doctor's office through MyChart or by email ahead of your next appointment. You may or may not get a reply, but at least you will have gotten your questions on the table for discussion. Consider taking notes when you meet with your doctor, unless they give you clear written instructions at the end of your appointment.

TAKING CONTROL STRATEGY 3: Take a trusted family member or friend with you to your psychiatry sessions

When you engage your support people in learning about each medicine, they may think of questions that hadn't occurred to you. They may be able to coach you on how to address your concerns with the doctor. You will probably need to clear their attendance at sessions with your doctor, but most will be OK with it as long as they also have some individual time with you.

TAKING CONTROL STRATEGY 4: Bring your therapist into the loop

If you're seeing a nonphysician therapist (for example, a psychologist or social worker), it's important to let them know what medications you're taking—including those prescribed by your GP for other medical reasons—and the name of your prescribing physician. Then encourage communication between this therapist and your physician(s) via signing release-of-information forms. Ideally, your providers work as a team, with periodic contact to monitor your overall progress. Therapists may be the first to notice a side effect and bring it to your and your doctor's attention (hand tremors being one example).

You may be tempted to ask your therapist questions about your medications, especially if you're comfortable with them or your psychiatrist is hard to reach. Although your therapist may be quite knowledgeable about medicines, they will probably refer you back to your prescriber for answers.

Coping with Daily Problems with Medications

"I'm having trouble staying on my meds. How do I figure out whether I'm having side effects or the meds just aren't improving my symptoms? It's like the treatment is worse than the disease."

It's one thing to agree to take medications after one or two episodes, but how about over time? Many people with BD start off taking mood stabilizers or antipsychotics but then go off them or take them inconsistently. The table on the facing page lists some of the common problems people have in sticking with their medications and some of the things they can do (with the help of physician and family supports) to make medications more manageable.

Daily Problems with Medications and Their Solutions

Problem area	What can you do?	How can your family help?
"My medications cost too much."	Ask your physician about generics. If you're paying for two (or more) pills of the same drug to achieve the desired dose, ask the prescriber if there is a way to write for a higher dose of a single pill to minimize multiple copays for different doses. Also, check drug coupon sites like *www.goodrx.com*.	Offer financial help; communicate with your insurance provider.
"My medications have stopped working (or never worked in the first place)."	Define your optimal state of wellness/recovery (such as ratings of –1 (*mild depression*) to +1 (*mild hypomania*) on your mood chart). Then plot when you started or stopped different medications. What is the evidence that no medications have worked, or that certain medications have improved your moods whereas others haven't?	Get feedback from your family members; ask them whether they think one agent (or regimen) has worked better than others.
"I see no reason to take medications if I'm well and have no symptoms."	Consider that mood stabilizers and antipsychotics are preventive medications that reduce the likelihood of future episodes and their severity.	If you have a partner or close friend who is good at judging your emotional state, ask them if they think you are symptom-free.
"I can control my illness without medications."	Ask yourself whether this has been true historically; how have you managed to control your illness in the past?	Get a second opinion from a trusted relative or friend: Are you in control of your mood states now, or have you been in the past? Were medications helpful at those times?
"Meds leave me feeling blunted and emotionless, and resentful that my moods are being controlled."	Talk to your doctor about whether dosages can be adjusted to allow you more mood variability.	Ask your relatives or friends: Do I seem flat/boring/zoned out? Am I not as funny as I used to be? Does it seem like my personality has changed?
"I can't remember to take my meds"; "I always miss my morning dose."	Consider pillboxes, Smartphone apps, and automated reminders. Pair taking your meds with daily routines like breakfast; discuss once-a-day dosing with your doctor.	Ask family members to remind you or suggest ways you can remind yourself, without being intrusive.

TAKING CONTROL STRATEGY 1: Discuss with your doctor strategies to minimize side effects

Medical management of side effects usually involves one of the following:

- Changing the dosage
- Using divided dosages (taking a medication more than once a day if a single dose produces many side effects, for example)
- Taking with food to minimize nausea
- Changing to a single daily dose, usually to reduce forgetting or in some cases to reduce side effects
- Changing to nighttime dosing to reduce sedation
- Gradually going off of one medication and introducing a different agent (a "cross-taper")
- Adding a second mood stabilizer, antipsychotic, or antidepressant if the first one isn't working adequately
- Adding agents that are meant specifically for side effects (Metformin for weight management; amiloride for excessive urination from lithium)

Just as one example, if lithium makes you feel emotionally flat or less creative, you can discuss with your doctor lowering the dosage so that you can experience more mood variability without having full episodes. Another example: physical restlessness and motor slowing, which are common side effects of antipsychotics, can be controlled with dosage reductions or sometimes by adding medicines, like beta blockers for restlessness or anticholinergic medications (such as benztropine) for motor slowing. The sexual side effects of serotonin reuptake inhibitors (SSRIs) like Prozac—such as reduced sexual drive or male impotence—can often be addressed by lowering dosages or switching to antidepressants that have different mechanisms of action, such as bupropion (Wellbutrin) or vilazodone (Viibryd).

TAKING CONTROL STRATEGY 2: Keep your own medical record

It can be very helpful to keep a journal of information about medicines you have taken, your doses, and their individual effects and side effects (good or bad), as well as copies of pertinent lab reports (for example, lithium levels) and results of psychological testing. When you consult a new doctor who asks whether you've tried drug X, being able to refer to this record can feel empowering.

"My doctor has tried changing my medications and lowering doses, but my side effects don't go away. What else can I do?"

TAKING CONTROL STRATEGY: Be realistic about the pros and cons of medications

Some of the problems with medicines can't be solved by simply adjusting dosages or switching to a different agent, and the process of adjusting and readjusting can be incredibly frustrating. Often people in this position start thinking about doing without medications entirely. If you find yourself wondering whether you could do without them, or whether you could control your moods with simple lifestyle adjustments like sleep, think through the pros and cons. Yes, you may be relieved of shaking hands, weight gain, sedation, or sexual side effects, all of which can impair your quality of life, but stopping medications altogether can also mean risking having a new episode. An abundance of research suggests that suddenly stopping mood stabilizers or antidepressants can lead to mood recurrences or even suicidal behavior. Having a recurrence of mania or depression or a renewed phase of cycling between hypomania and depression can impair your quality of life in even more dramatic ways than side effects.

If you're unhappy with your regimen—whether due to side effects, costs, or uncertainty about whether a drug is effective—be proactive and discuss your concerns with your doctor to see if there is a better solution than just stopping them. Your doctor should be open to helping you find personalized solutions to complaints like the ones in the table on page 215. Discuss alternatives to the medications you're taking, which may include strategies you haven't tried yet, such as specific forms of psychotherapy (Chapter 14), light therapy, new medicines for severe depression (such as ketamine), or TMS.

 "The social stigma of taking psychiatric medications is enough to make me not want to take them."

Many people feel their medications make them appear physically debilitated, awkward, or slow. Taking meds can feel tantamount to admitting you are mentally ill, impaired, or dangerous, which can make you want to stop them completely. Indeed, physical side effects can be a source of questions from others, including potential romantic partners. These are very real issues for people with BD. How do you explain these things to other people?

TAKING CONTROL STRATEGY 1: Be up-front with people

If you're dating someone new (or you have a new employer) and they ask you about your shaking hands, why you sometimes seem slowed down, or why you've canceled evenings out or missed work, this is a good time to educate them about what medications you take and why. Lay out your regimen for them in a factual way— why and for how long you've been taking them, what side effects they cause, and what strategies you use to manage them. Sometimes this is best done when you first disclose your diagnosis (see Chapter 8), but it depends on who you want to tell and why. Consult the recommendations in Chapter 9 regarding how to ask for work accommodations or work release time for medical visits.

TAKING CONTROL STRATEGY 2: Frame medications for mood disorders as similar to medications for any physical illness

In the same way that comparing BD to physical disorders can help destigmatize it, so can making comparisons with medications used for common physical ailments. For example, antihypertensives (to reduce blood pressure) can, like SSRIs, interfere with sexual performance. Drugs used for managing migraine headaches can be associated with mental sluggishness or dullness.

Most people with BD have one or more nonpsychiatric physical illnesses for which they take medicine. It can be hard to tell whether a suspected side effect is caused by a psychiatric drug, a nonpsychiatric drug, or an interaction between drugs—all things to discuss with your doctor.

TAKING CONTROL STRATEGY 3: Be aware of self-talk

As you know, strong feelings about how others see us often reflect feelings about ourselves. It's important to be aware of self-talk associated with medications and how those thoughts make you feel, such as "When I take lithium, I feel like I'm a defective person"; "I look stupid or awkward on Risperdal"; or "No one will want to go out with me now that I've gained so much weight on Zyprexa." Such self-doubts are understandable, but medications and illness labels do not define you. You have not fundamentally changed; your strengths and abilities are still there. Combat these thoughts with self-statements like "I'm a person with bipolar disorder, I'm not 'a bipolar'"; "People take medications for many different things; they don't change who you are as a person"; and "Lots of people have trouble with their weight, and for lots of different reasons." You may not believe these self-statements at first, but acknowledging your self-doubts and rehearsing counterthoughts is an essential coping strategy.

Your Family and Your Medications: Odd Bedfellows?

 "My family is always pushing me to take more pills or asking me whether I've taken them today. It makes me want to stop taking them altogether."

Family members can be of considerable help in dealing with the day-to-day problems caused by your treatments. But as you saw in the table on page 127, well-meaning family members can also contribute to discouragement regarding medications. When a parent or spouse is constantly nagging you to take more or a different type of medicine, reminding you, or checking on your side effects, you will feel like you are a patient rather than a relative. You can feel stigmatized within your own family if every time you get angry or emotional about something, you are asked whether you've taken your pills that day. Here's an example scenario:

> Julia, age 19, was taking valproate (Depakote) and quetiapine (Seroquel) following a severe, hospitalized manic episode. As she began to recover, she still had residual symptoms, such as talking loudly and out of turn. At Thanksgiving dinner when talking to her cousins, she became quite excited and animated during a debate about climate change. She enjoyed the stimulating back-and-forth, until, during a brief gap in the conversation, she heard her grandmother say, "Is she still taking her pills?" She began to cry and abruptly left the table.

TAKING CONTROL STRATEGY 1: Develop a shared framework for when, how often, and in what context your family members can discuss medications with you

Make sure your conversations with family members aren't always focused on your medications. You can tell them the following:

> "It's not a good idea to keep asking me about my medicines. Instead, talk to me about the things that have happened in my life (and in yours) in a collaborative way. If you want to bring up medicines once in a while, fine, but don't make it the basis of all our conversations."

Relatedly, explain how you feel when they bring up the topic when others are around. These conversations are best had before visitors come over, the same way you might ask your parents not to bring up a recent relationship breakup or job loss.

TAKING CONTROL STRATEGY 2: Show your independence by filling your own prescriptions, making doctor appointments, and dealing with your insurance

The more personal agency you show in dealing with your health care, the less your family members will bug you.

 "My parents (spouse) think I should stop taking medications. They keep telling me I'm just going through something hormonal. They just don't get it."

TAKING CONTROL STRATEGY: Express your independence regarding medication-related decisions

It's best to avoid control battles over your use of medications. Family members may oppose your use of them based on their own negative experiences with doctors, their prior reactions to medications, or their belief that your mood swings have some other (nonpsychiatric) cause. Although you can listen to and express an understanding of their opinions, make clear that these decisions are yours and should come out of a working relationship between you and your doctor. Here is an example of how to set limits:

FATHER: You don't need those drugs. They're a crutch.

YOU: I know you feel that way, Dad, but I think of these things differently.

FATHER: What good will they do? Life is full of stress. You can't just make everything go away with pills.

YOU: I understand, but as you know, I have a mood disorder that makes dealing with stress much different than it might be for you. You'll have to trust my judgment about my health care. I feel like I'm in good hands with Dr. _____. I'd appreciate your support on my decisions, or at least not to push back on me, which just adds more stress.

FATHER: Why don't you see one of those hormone specialists to get a second opinion?

YOU: I will consider that, especially if my psychiatrist recommends it. But right now, this is the direction I'm going to take. Now, let's talk about something else.

Taking Stock

Once you've equipped yourself with enough information about your medicines and the process of pharmacological treatment, try to complete the self-assessment in the form on page 222 so that you know where you stand. Revisit these questions from time to time, as your answers may change with experience. You can even hand this completed form to a family member who is bugging you about your treatment, especially when you find yourself getting annoyed or tongue-tied.

A Word about Acceptance

Learning to cope with your medications is a moving target. The pills you're taking now may not be the same ones you take next year, or even a few months from now. Always give your medications enough time to work before stopping or changing them. Never stop your medications suddenly, which for some prescriptions (particularly lithium, but also antidepressants) can precipitate a recurrence. If you're determined to stop, discuss the process of tapering with your doctor—there are right and wrong ways to do it.

The hardest adjustment comes with time: accepting the discomforts that come with BD and the medicines that treat it. The side effects can be maddening, as can the societal stigma, but you're trading these misfortunes for a more stable life and a healthier economic, practical, and emotional outlook. If this seems like a raw deal, reopen the conversation with your doctor and see what adjustments can be made. If you're still not satisfied, get a second opinion. You should not have to compromise on leading a balanced and fulfilling life.

SELF-ASSESSMENT
OF MEDICATION REGIMENS

What medications are now being recommended, and at what dosage?

_____   _____

_____   _____

_____   _____

What is your understanding of why they're being recommended?

Do you agree with these recommendations? If not, recount your reasons
for not wanting to take one or all of them.

What do you see as the risks of not taking them?

If you are taking them regularly, what side effects do you experience?

What have you learned about dealing with side effects?

How are your family members or spouse communicating with you about
your meds? Is it helping or not? What would you want to be different?

14

psychosocial treatment

LIVING WELL WHILE MAINTAINING MOOD STABILITY

Having the right medications, making lifestyle adjustments (like keeping regular sleep/wake cycles), and having regular evidence-based psychotherapy are the three elements of optimal care for BD. This is true regardless of your age, whether you're having your first episode or have had many, you have bipolar I or II, or any number of other variations. Unfortunately, once people with BD achieve mood stability with medications, many decide they don't need further treatment, in the same way they might forget about their teeth between dental appointments. Yet there is plenty of evidence that regular psychotherapy can reduce your symptoms and improve your quality of life above and beyond medications.

Psychosocial treatment (my preferred term over *psychotherapy*, the latter of which has Freudian overtones) is recommended as *an add-on* to medications, not as a substitute. It can help you make progress on issues that medication can't touch: your feelings about having BD, the quality of your intimate relationships, your functioning on the job, your experiences of stigma, how to get along with your family members or achieve stability in your marriage, the impact of traumatic experiences or adversity in child- or adulthood, and how to find meaning and satisfaction in life despite the illness. Some of these issues improve when your symptoms improve, but some do not, or they might not improve to the extent that you would wish. In this chapter you'll learn about how the types of therapy available for BD can improve your daily life and how to find the best therapy (and therapist) for your individual needs.

 "What will I talk about in therapy, and how will the therapist help me? I don't want them to just nod their head and say, 'You'll be OK.'"

Many people with BD swear by psychosocial treatment and consider it life-saving (see, for example, Kay Jamison's [1995] account in *An Unquiet Mind*). Others are disappointed, viewing it as a waste of time and an expensive way to maintain a friendship. Given its biological and genetic causes, why do people with BD need therapy as well as medications? What kinds of problems do they talk about?

TAKING CONTROL STRATEGY: Know what kinds of help are available

The table on pages 225–226 lists the kinds of issues that routinely come up for people with BD (and in other recurrent psychiatric disorders) that can wreck one's daily life. The table also illustrates how different therapies would go about solving (or at least fostering insight into) these problems. You may find it helpful to high-light or circle any problems that resonate with you, which may help narrow down the therapy that will help you most.

An unfortunate caveat is that not all of these psychosocial treatments will be available in your community. Some can be obtained online (through Zoom or another telehealth platform) from major universities or medical centers, and some may be available in your community after a waiting period. Nonetheless, if you can find a good provider who offers one of these treatments and stick with it long enough (generally, at least 12 sessions), you will be at lower risk for recurrences and have an easier time dealing with stressors that evoke episodes.

 "My therapy has been endless and doesn't seem to be leading anywhere. How do I get on the same page with my therapist?"

Many people find individual therapy helpful at the beginning and then reach a point of diminishing returns. If you sense this is happening, discuss it with your therapist.

TAKING CONTROL STRATEGY 1: Review your initial goals with your therapist and make the timeline explicit

Common Problems in BD and How They Are Addressed in Psychosocial Treatment

Problem	Psychosocial treatment strategies	Type of therapy
"I'm struggling with accepting that I have BD. It feels like a roadblock, and it's causing conflict with my family. What am I missing?"	Psychoeducation for you and your spouse/family members about what is and isn't a symptom of BD (e.g., being happy is not the same as being manic); facilitating communication about your and their beliefs about the disorder; addressing your feelings about psychiatric medications.	Family-focused therapy (conducted conjointly with at least one of your family members) or family support groups (with other families)
"My parents are extremely critical of me. They think if I just take more pills I'll be able to finish school and reach my potential. It makes me want to fight them by just quitting all my meds. They don't seem to understand what I can and can't do with this disorder."	Educate your parents about how BD can affect your life goals and achievements; practice collaborative communication strategies with them, such as diplomatic requests for behavior change and problem solving, so that they don't rely on criticism or nagging.	Family-focused therapy
"I start thinking about how, if I just stopped all my medications and went back to doing the things I did before I got ill, everything would go well for me."	Explore "grieving the lost self," the tendency to think about one's life as divided into the periods before and after you became ill; obtain help in revising your goals to take into account the limitations imposed by the illness.	Interpersonal and social rhythm therapy
"My interactions with specific people (such as my boss and certain coworkers) trigger my mood swings. I can barely make it through the day."	Explore how your moods affect interpersonal relationships and how these relationships affect your moods; consider alternative interpretations of the causes of your own or others' behavior.	Interpersonal and social rhythm therapy or cognitive-behavioral therapy
"I haven't been successful in finding a romantic relationship. I date someone for a few months and then it ends."	Explore interpersonal habits, styles of communication, or thinking patterns that may be affecting relationships—and whether these habits are affected by your mood states.	Interpersonal and social rhythm therapy or cognitive-behavioral therapy
"I need help with balance—how to organize my life so that I sleep well and don't get thrown by small changes in my routines."	Work toward keeping regulated sleep/wake habits and daily/nightly routines; anticipate those events that dysregulate routines and implement self-regulation strategies.	Interpersonal and social rhythm therapy *(continued)*

Note. Some of these problems are addressed in multiple forms of psychosocial treatment. For example, keeping regular sleep/wake hours is a recommendation of nearly all therapies. The therapy listed after each problem area is the one that is most clearly designed to address it.

Common Problems in BD (*continued*)

Problem	Psychosocial treatment strategies	Type of therapy
"I feel very alone with my illness. How can I find other people who have gone through the same things?"	Meet with other people with BD to share experiences with the disorder and coping strategies.	Mutual support groups (with psychoeducational framework); may be available for family members separately
"I have these really intense periods of rage and self-hatred. When I feel worst, I start thinking about suicide, I try to cut myself, or I get hopelessly drunk and self-destructive."	Learn distress tolerance, emotion regulation, and mindfulness skills to manage your reactions when in an emotional crisis.	Dialectical behavior therapy, often combining group and individual skill-training sessions
"I feel like my negative thinking gets in the way of enjoying things. Even when good things happen I overemphasize the terrible things that could have gone wrong."	Explore self-talk about the causes of certain events, along with predictions about the future; challenge these predictions and consider alternative ways of thinking.	Cognitive-behavioral therapy
"I can't seem to get out of my depression—I'm stuck, with long periods of time just lying in bed."	Practice behavioral activation exercises in which a therapist guides you in making small daily advances in your physical and social activity; engage family members in helping achieve your daily goals.	Cognitive-behavioral therapy, combined with family-focused therapy sessions as relevant
"I love my manic periods—they're exciting and full of life. I get bored by daily life, and then I want to stop my meds."	Explore how you could find excitement and stimulation without stopping your meds; evaluate your assumptions about how life will go without them.	Group psychoeducation; cognitive-behavioral therapy
"When my depression gets worse, I start drinking heavily, and then everything deteriorates."	Employ harm reduction approaches to substance use; reduce the triggers for craving and use.	Cognitive-behavioral and motivational enhancement approaches; "dual-diagnosis" drug abuse/bipolar groups

As with any service you're paying for, you deserve to know how long it will take and how you will know when the job is done. Ideally, at the beginning of therapy, define your goals with your therapist and how you will both monitor your progress. If the goal is "learning to cope with mood symptoms," how will you and your therapist determine when you've achieved this goal? If the goal is "having better relationships" (a rather broad objective), what is the treatment plan to move in this direction?

You may be thinking, "Isn't this the therapist's job, to keep clarifying my goals and reviewing my progress?" Yes, but your therapist may be thinking about your treatment quite differently from you. For example, they may see treatment planning as still in the development stage when you think problems should have been solved by now. In any case, if you have concerns, it's always better to bring them up.

TAKING CONTROL STRATEGY 2: Discuss booster sessions with your therapist

Psychosocial treatment can be a slow process, and change can be hard to achieve in short periods of time. Nonetheless, it shouldn't go on forever. If you've been in individual therapy for more than a couple of months, sessions may take on an automated quality, where you talk about your week, your therapist asks about your mood and provides a few clarifications or suggestions, and off you go. If this is occurring, pose some questions to your clinician: Do they think you're improving, and in what way? What would they hope you'll achieve in the next 3 months? Does it make sense to continue? Be prepared to answer these questions from your vantage point, because inevitably your therapist will ask for your opinions on these matters.

If you've had a good experience with a particular therapist and don't want to stop but no longer need to meet every week, discuss the possibility of meeting every other week or even meeting for *booster sessions* every few months. These less frequent (or shorter) sessions can be a reasonable compromise if you have not had any major symptoms or other upheavals for a while. Booster sessions may keep you attuned to triggers in your social, work, or family life that, historically, have precipitated new episodes (for example, major changes in sleep/wake hours; significant family, relationship, or job conflicts; a new romantic relationship) and that are amenable to prevention plans.

TAKING CONTROL STRATEGY 3: Explore whether the treatment plan needs to be modified

It's not usually a good idea to just quit your therapy and hope you'll find a better clinician. Instead, try to explore your options with the therapist systematically, including the option of revising the treatment plan. For example, you may want to talk less about current moods or stressors and more about traumatic events in childhood. Perhaps you have comorbid ADHD and want to develop strategies to improve your attention and concentration. You may want to talk more about your relationship with your partner or include them in conjoint sessions. Your therapist

may be open to making these shifts or refer you to another provider who special-
izes in these issues.

TAKING CONTROL STRATEGY 4: Get another opinion

As with your psychiatrist, you may benefit from hearing the opinions of another
psychological therapist. Your therapist should be able to refer you to other clinicians in your community. If you live in a rural or suburban setting, there may be
options for therapy from specialists through telehealth.

 **"I've seen therapists who claim to know all about BD, and I feel
like I've given them a fair chance. But I don't feel like they've
really helped me. How do I find the right one?"**

TAKING CONTROL STRATEGY 1: Locate a therapist who routinely treats people with BD and understands the need for communication with your medical prescriber

Locating the right therapist is often the hardest part of getting effective treatment.
Few therapists have a specialty in BD (unless they're connected with a larger clinical or research program, usually based in medical schools). Worse yet, some claim
to be experts but really have no idea how to treat people with BD, seeing it as just
an extension of depression or the result of childhood trauma. Some may try to convince you that you have a different illness, even though you've had your diagnosis
verified by multiple providers. Here are some online resources and lists of clinicians
who report training in BD:

> International Bipolar Foundation: *https://ibpf.org/learn/resources*
> International Society for Bipolar Disorders: *www.isbd.org/Global_resources*
> Association for Behavioral and Cognitive Therapies: *https://services.abct.org/
> i4a/memberDirectory/index.cfm*

Although you may locate some relevant names or programs through these
sites, you'll have to talk to each provider directly to determine whether they are
trained in one of the therapies described above, or whether they practice novel (and
hopefully research-based) assessment or treatment strategies. Their online listing
doesn't imply endorsement by the organization.

Regardless of whether the therapist has a specialization in BD, they should be
collaborating with the person prescribing your medications. They may or may not
know this prescriber, but they should at least agree to talk with the prescriber on a

semi-regular basis (at least once every couple of months) to monitor your progress and exchange information about your responses to medications and therapy. They should know enough about the medications you take to be able to recognize side effects.

TAKING CONTROL STRATEGY 2: Assess the "fit" of a new therapist

When vetting a new therapist, your decision on whether to continue should be based in part on whether you and they are a good fit. Your assessment should be based in part on their responses to your questions and in part on your gut feeling about whether you should work with them. Here's an example:

> Alice, age 23, had been through three lengthy depressive episodes and at least two periods of hypomania, one of which was fueled by the drug ecstasy. She had been diagnosed with bipolar II disorder by three different psychiatrists. During a first psychosocial treatment session, her new therapist asked her a few questions about her mood symptoms but focused mainly on her drug use and relationships with men. At the end of the session the therapist pronounced, "You don't have bipolar disorder. You're depressed and have problems with drugs. You probably need to take an antidepressant." When Alice pressed her on why she didn't believe Alice had BD—and how therapy would help—the therapist said, "We need to figure out why you always choose destructive relationships." Alice was turned off by the therapist's approach and did not go back.

As you can see from this brief vignette, the fit between Alice's experiences and the therapist's approach was wrong. Here are some clues that may suggest the therapist is not a good fit: they say they don't deal much with BD; they opine that it's "usually the wrong diagnosis," preferring to diagnose posttraumatic stress disorder, personality disorders, ADHD, or just depression; or they say that BD is really only treated with medicines, with a minimal role for therapy. Depending on where you live, your economic situation, and your insurance plan, you should look for another provider.

Some people feel strongly that the clinician should have a doctoral or medical degree (MD), but that is not as important as the person's training and experience level. There is no evidence that people seeing a well-trained social worker (for example) have any lesser outcome than those who see a well-trained psychologist or psychiatrist. The personality fit with the clinician—such as the feeling that they genuinely care about you—is far more important than their degree.

TAKING CONTROL STRATEGY 3: Explain to the therapist what outcome you would like to achieve

How do your individual goals align with the therapist's? If you have just met the therapist and told them your story, what do they say about their initial goals for you? What will be the focus—your BD and its effects on your life, current or past life stressors or trauma, family or romantic relationships, functioning on the job, feelings of stigma? your patterns of self-talk, interpersonal habits, or feelings about taking medications? It may take a few sessions before the clinician can answer these questions effectively, so give them a chance.

TAKING CONTROL STRATEGY 4: Determine if the therapist is aligned with the approaches that we know to be effective in BD

Most of the evidence-based therapies listed in the table on pages 225–226 have a psychoeducational focus, meaning they are oriented toward helping you understand and cope with BD: how to anticipate and deal with triggers for mood episodes, adopt lifestyle management strategies (such as mindfulness meditation for coping with anxiety and depression, tracking your symptoms, and early warning signs, or practicing communication skills), gain control over substance or alcohol abuse, and make use of the mental health system. When discussing treatment goals related to your BD, can the therapist go beyond "We want to get you more stable"?

 "What form of therapy—individual, group, or family/couple—is best for me?"

TAKING CONTROL STRATEGY 1: Figure out whether you are comfortable in support groups

Some treatments are conducted in groups with other people who have BD. There is evidence that group and family formats for psychoeducation may be more effective in preventing illness recurrences than individual therapy formats in BD. Group treatments with other individuals with BD enable you to see how others cope with the disorder and not feel so alone in your struggles. You can be fairly certain that others in the group have struggled with social stigma, navigating the mental health system, ambiguity about which medications to take, and relationship or family problems related to the illness.

Not everyone is comfortable in group therapy. You may feel uncomfortable about exploring private matters with strangers, whose willingness to keep your personal information confidential may not feel reliable. You may worry that others will scoff at your concerns. You may find yourself in a group with much older or younger individuals whose problems don't resemble your own, or with members who can't stop talking about themselves. Usually, you can try out a group one or two times before committing to it. If the composition is right, you may be surprised at how supportive it feels.

Group therapy for BD is usually structured with a leader who is a trained clinician (usually a psychologist or social worker) who directs the group in skill-oriented exercises, such as agreeing on ways to cope with medication side effects, constructing a list of early warning signs or learning to navigate stigmatizing situations. Alternatively, the leader may be a "peer counselor": an individual with BD who has been trained to help others. These kinds of groups are usually provided for free by the Depression and Bipolar Support Alliance (*www.dbsalliance.org/support*) or the National Alliance on Mental Illness (*www.nami.org/Support-Education/Support-Groups*) along with other community mental health organizations.

TAKING CONTROL STRATEGY 2: Weigh the pros and cons of having your parents or partner involved in treatment

FFT, the 4- to 6-month treatment my team and I developed at the University of California, Los Angeles (UCLA) and the University of Colorado, is effective in preventing recurrences and reducing the severity of mood symptoms in people with BD; there are also benefits for your family or marital relationships. If you can find a provider who works with families of people with BD—whether or not they have formal training in FFT—you may be able to accomplish some or all of the following:

- Educate your family about your early warning signs for depressive or manic episodes, and how to be supportive when you're going into an episode or coming off of one.
- Recalibrating their expectations when your cognitive functioning is impaired during or after an episode.
- Learn and practice skills for communicating and solving problems related to the illness and family life (such as how to talk about medications; how they can express their expectations of you without criticism).
- Clear up misunderstandings about your motives (such as a parent's accusation that you are not trying hard enough) or about how your personality attributes differ from your mood symptoms.
- Get relatives on your side in communicating with your physician or other relevant providers.

Family therapy with one's parents or siblings is not, of course, for everyone. First, it can be difficult to talk about your disorder with family members present, especially if you feel acute resentment about how they've treated you during current or past episodes. Some parents refuse to be involved because they fear being blamed for causing your illness, either through their parenting or through the genes they passed on. There is a long and unfortunate history in mental health care of placing the blame on parents for various kinds of emotional problems in their offspring. A good family therapist will make it clear that they do not hold anyone responsible for having caused the illness.

If your relatives want to learn about your disorder but you can't find a suitable family therapist—or you or they don't want to do therapy together—there are groups for relatives, such as the Family-to-Family program of the National Alliance on Mental Illness (*www.nami.org/Support-Education/Mental-Health-Education/NAMI-Family-to-Family*) or the For Friends and Family support groups of the Depression and Bipolar Support Alliance (*www.dbsalliance.org/support/for-friends-family*).

TAKING CONTROL STRATEGY 3: Locate a good family or couple therapist

Family and couple therapy involve a specific set of techniques that not all clinicians are trained in providing. Look for local options for family therapists by searching on *https://match.talkspace.com/flow/90/step/1* or the American Association for Marriage and Family Therapy's website (*www.aamft.org/directories/find_a_therapist.aspx*) or Psychology Today's therapist location pages (*www.psychologytoday.com/us/therapists*). Then, narrow the search to one or more clinicians who have some experience with BD, rather than starting by finding a bipolar expert.

Family and couple therapy can be done online, which has the advantage that you and your spouse or family members don't have to travel long distances for what amounts to a 1-hour session.

Be thorough in vetting your family or couple therapist: They vary considerably in terms of skill, training, and experience (not to mention cost). You can interview them by phone before you make a commitment. Ask them how often they have worked with people with BD in a family or couple context, how they usually proceed, and whether they will be in regular contact with your prescriber.

An Example of FFT

Karla was 18 and in her senior year of high school. After the onset of a depressive episode, she began sessions of FFT with two older siblings (a biological sister and stepbrother) and her biological mother and stepfather. The clinician began by obtaining Karla's agreement to discuss her bipolar diagnosis with her family members and encouraged her parents and siblings to share their observations about her symptoms. The family members differed in their explanations of Karla's depression: childhood trauma, inheritance, stress, "laziness," or (in the words of her older brother), "hormones, probably." Karla also described clear periods of increased energy, irritability, impulsive behavior, decreased sleep, and hypersexuality, none of which had been apparent to her family members. She felt disengaged from her family, saying, "everyone just goes about doing their own thing."

Karla and her family members held different opinions on whether she needed medications. Karla expressed fear that "there's something wrong with my brain—maybe it's broken" and that taking a pill would ruin her chances of getting into a good college. Her mother wanted her to try Lexapro (escitalopram), but hadn't considered the possibility that antidepressants might not be the first recommendation for a person with BD. Her stepfather expressed concern about addiction to psychiatric drugs, which the clinician explained was not a concern with mood stabilizers or antipsychotics.

The clinician encouraged Karla's family members to share their own experiences of treatment for depression; indeed, her mother and older sister had both had depressive episodes and had received SSRIs and therapy. This discussion made Karla feel less stigmatized, a key issue behind her questions about her broken brain. Karla's stepfather found the discussion especially useful, given his assumption that she was being lazy and didn't really want to go to college. Karla eventually agreed to an evaluation with a psychiatrist and began a trial of lamotrigine.

The majority of the FFT sessions focused on exchanges in which each member practiced open and effective communication: being able to listen to one another's expressions of emotional pain or confusion, learning how to request changes in one another's behavior (such as avoiding yelling when frustrated), and balancing negative feedback or criticism with praise. At the end of the 4-month treatment, Karla's depression had lifted; she remained on lamotrigine and was actively applying to colleges. The family reported a greater understanding of her BD and that their communication had become more honest and direct.

Taking Stock

Many people say that their psychosocial treatment is just as important as their medications. But it has to be with the right therapist dealing with issues that are relevant to your life as well as your disorder. When choosing a therapist, take your time to see what they have to offer. It can be a long-term commitment, and it makes sense to choose wisely if you have options, even if that means therapist shopping for a while.

Be an informed consumer when it comes to getting what you need from therapy. Good therapy should give you a better understanding of your disorder, as well as teach you ways to improve your relationships, deal with stress, implement lifestyle adjustments, and function well in school or on the job. Sometimes, what you address in therapy will be directly relevant to your disorder (or comorbid disorders like ADHD) and at other times will be entirely separate. Therapy may wax and wane in its efficacy over time, but it's critical that you and your therapist be on the same page about your goals.

If your therapist and psychiatrist work as a team, with regular communication, it's like having a second family that cares enough about you to make sure your treatment is optimal. In the words of Kay Jamison, "Psychotherapy . . . is where I have believed—or have learned to believe—that I might someday be able to contend with all of this" (*An Unquiet Mind,* 1995, pages 88–89).

bibliography

Introduction

Miklowitz, D. J. (2019). *The bipolar disorder survival guide: What you and your family need to know* (3rd ed.). New York: Guilford Press.

Part One

American Psychiatric Association. (2022). *Diagnostic and statistical manual of mental disorders* (5th ed., text rev.). Arlington, VA: Author.

Chapter 1

American Psychiatric Association. (2022). *Diagnostic and statistical manual of mental disorders* (5th ed., text rev.). Arlington, VA: Author.

Geddes, J. R., Calabrese, J. R., & Goodwin, G. M. (2009). Lamotrigine for treatment of bipolar depression: Independent meta-analysis and meta-regression of individual patient data from five randomised trials. *British Journal of Psychiatry, 194*(1), 4–9.

Teasdale, J., Williams, M., & Segal, Z. (2014). *The mindful way workbook: An 8-week program to free yourself from depression and emotional distress.* New York: Guilford Press.

Williams, M., Teasdale, J., Segal, Z., & Kabat-Zinn, J. (2007). *The mindful way through depression: Freeing yourself from chronic unhappiness.* New York: Guilford Press.

Williams, M., Teasdale, J., Segal, Z., & Kabat-Zinn, J. (in press). *The mindful way through depression: Freeing yourself from chronic unhappiness* (2nd ed.). New York: Guilford Press.

Zarate, C. A. J., Brutsche, N. E., Ibrahim, L., Franco-Chaves, J., Diazgranados, N., Cravchik, A., . . . Luckenbaugh, D. A. (2012). Replication of ketamine's antidepressant efficacy in bipolar depression: A randomized controlled add-on trial. *Biological Psychiatry, 71*(11), 939–946.

Chapter 3

Wagner, A. P. (2002). *Worried no more: Help and hope for anxious children.* Lighthouse Point, FL: Lighthouse Press.

Chapter 4

Garrett, A. S., Armstrong, C., Chang, K. D., Singh, M. K., Walshaw, P. D., & Miklowitz, D. J. (2021). Neural changes in youth at high risk for bipolar disorder undergoing family-focused therapy or psychoeducation. *Bipolar Disorders, 23*(6), 604–614.

Strakowski, S. M., Adler, C. M., Almeida, J., Altshuler, L. L., Blumberg, H. P., Chang, K. D., . . . Townsend, J. D. (2012). The functional neuroanatomy of bipolar disorder: A consensus model. *Bipolar Disorders, 14*(4), 313–325.

Williams, J. M. G., & Penman, D. (2011). *Mindfulness: An 8-week plan for finding peace in a frantic world.* Emmaus, PA: Rodale Books.

Chapter 5

Hooley, J. M., & Franklin, J. C. (2018). Why do people hurt themselves? A new conceptual model of nonsuicidal self-injury. *Clinical Psychological Science, 6,* 428–451.

Jamison, K. R. (2000). *Night falls fast: Understanding suicide.* New York: Vintage Books.

Kiekens, G., Claes, L., Hasking, P., Mortier, P., Bootsma, E., Boyes, M., . . . Bruffaerts, R. (2023). A longitudinal investigation of non-suicidal self-injury persistence patterns, risk factors, and clinical outcomes during the college period. *Psychological Medicine, 53*(13), 6011–6026.

Solomon, A. (2002). *Noonday demon: An atlas of depression.* New York: Scribner.

Styron, W. (1992). *Darkness visible: A memoir of madness.* New York: Vintage Books.

Wilkinson, S. T., Trujillo Diaz, D., Rupp, Z. W., Kidambi, A., Ramirez, K. L., Flores, J. M., . . . Bloch, M. H. (2023). Pharmacological and somatic treatment effects on suicide in adults: A systematic review and meta-analysis. *Focus, 21*(2), 197–208.

Chapter 6

Carney, C. E., Buysse, D. J., Ancoli-Israel, S., Edinger, J. D., Krystal, A. D., Lichstein, K. L., & Morin, C. M. (2012). The consensus sleep diary: Standardizing prospective sleep self-monitoring. *Sleep, 35*(2), 287–302.

Giglio, L. M., Magalhaes, P. V., Andersen, M. L., Walz, J. C., Jakobson, L., & Kapczinski, F. (2010). Circadian preference in bipolar disorder. *Sleeping and Breathing, 14*(2), 153–155.

Gruber, J., Harvey, A. G., Wang, P. W., Brooks, J. O., 3rd, Thase, M. E., Sachs, G. S., & Ketter, T. A. (2009). Sleep functioning in relation to mood, function, and quality of life at entry to the Systematic Treatment Enhancement Program for Bipolar Disorder (STEP-BD). *Journal of Affective Disorders, 114*(1–3), 41–49.

Kaplan, K. A., Talavera, D. C., & Harvey, A. G. (2018). Rise and shine: A treatment experiment testing a morning routine to decrease subjective sleep inertia in insomnia and bipolar disorder. *Behavior Research and Therapy, 111,* 106–112.

Ohayon, M. M., Mahowald, M. W., & Leger, D. (2014). Are confusional arousals pathological? *Neurology, 83*(9), 834–841.

Soreca, I., Levenson, J., Lotz, M., Frank, E., & Kupfer, D. J. (2012). Sleep apnea risk and clinical correlates in patients with bipolar disorder. *Bipolar Disorders, 14*(6), 672–676.

Chapter 7

Cohen, M., Baker, G., Cohen, R. A., Fromm-Reichmann, F., & Weigert, V. (1954). An intensive study of 12 cases of manic-depressive psychosis. *Psychiatry, 17,* 103–137.

Miklowitz, D. J. (2007). The role of the family in the course and treatment of bipolar disorder. *Current Directions in Psychological Science, 16*(4), 192–196.

Miklowitz, D. J., Efthimiou, O., Furukawa, T. A., Scott, J., McLaren, R., Geddes, J. R., & Cipriani, A. (2021). Adjunctive psychotherapies for bipolar disorder: A systematic review and network meta-analysis. *JAMA Psychiatry, 78*(2), 141–150.

Sagar, K. A., Dahlgren, M. K., Gonenc, A., & Gruber, S. A. (2013). Altered affective processing in bipolar disorder: An fMRI study. *Journal of Affective Disorders, 150*(3), 1192–1196.

Wegbreit, E., Weissman, A. B., Cushman, G. K., Puzia, M. E., Kim, K. L., Leibenluft, E., & Dickstein, D. P. (2015). Facial emotion recognition in childhood-onset bipolar I disorder: An evaluation of developmental differences between youths and adults. *Bipolar Disorders, 17*(5), 471–485.

Chapter 8

Comfort, A. (2013). *The joy of sex: The ultimate revised edition.* New York: Harmony.

Jamison, K. R. (1995). *An unquiet mind: A memoir of moods and madness.* New York: Knopf.

Keck, P. E., Jr., McElroy, S. L., Strakowski, S. M., West, S. A., Sax, K. W., Hawkins, J. M., . . . Haggard, P. (1998). Twelve-month outcome of patients with bipolar disorder following hospitalization for a manic or mixed episode. *American Journal of Psychiatry, 155,* 646–652.

Rydahl, K. F. K., Brund, R. B. K., Medici, C. R., Straarup, K. M. N., Straszek, S. P. V., & Ostergaard, S. D. (2022). Bipolar disorder and regretted behavior in relation to use of social media and online dating. *Bipolar Disorders, 24*(1), 27–38.

Chapter 9

Gitlin, M. J., Mintz, J., Sokolski, K., Hammen, C., & Altshuler, L. L. (2011). Subsyndromal depressive symptoms after symptomatic recovery from mania are associated with delayed functional recovery. *Journal of Clinical Psychiatry, 72*(5), 692–697.

Iverson, G. L., Brooks, B. L., Langenecker, S. A., & Young, A. H. (2011). Identifying a cognitive impairment subgroup in adults with mood disorders. *Journal of Affective Disorders, 132*(3), 360–367.

Jamison, K. R. (1993). *Touched with fire: Manic-depressive illness and the artistic temperament.* New York: Macmillan International.

Loprinzi, P. D., Roig, M., Etnier, J. L., Tomporowski, P. D., & Voss, M. (2021). Acute and chronic exercise effects on human memory: What we know and where to go from here. *Journal of Clinical Medicine, 10*(21), 4812.

O'Donnell, L., Helmuth, M., Williams, S., McInnis, M. G., & Ryan, K. A. (2023). Predictors of employment status and stability in bipolar disorder: Findings from an 8-year longitudinal study. *Journal of Affective Disorders, 321,* 1–7.

Torres, I. J., Boudreau, V. G., & Yatham, L. N. (2007). Neuropsychological functioning in euthymic bipolar disorder: A meta-analysis. *Acta Psychiatrica Scandinavica Supplementum, 434,* 17–26.

U.S. Equal Employment Opportunity Commission. (1990). *The Americans with Disabilities Act of 1990, Titles I and V.* Washington, DC: Author. Accessed November 30, 2023, from *www.eeoc.gov/statutes/titles-i-and-v-americans-disabilities-act-1990-ada*

Ventriglio, A., Sancassiani, F., Contu, M. P., Latorre, M., Di Slavatore, M., Fornaro, M., & Bhugra, D. (2020). Mediterranean diet and its benefits on health and mental health: A literature review. *Clinical Practice and Epidemiology in Mental Health, 16*(Suppl. 1), 156–164.

Chapter 10

Bauer, I. E., Galvez, J. F., Hamilton, J. E., Balanza-Martinez, V., Zunta-Soares, G. B., Soares, J. C., & Meyer, T. D. (2016). Lifestyle interventions targeting dietary habits and exercise in bipolar disorder: A systematic review. *Journal of Psychiatric Research, 74*, 1–7.

Lewis, M. A., & Rook, K. S. (1999). Social control in personal relationships: Impact on health behaviors and psychological distress. *Health Psychology, 18*(1), 63–71.

Sylvia, L. G. (2015). *The wellness workbook for bipolar disorder: Your guide to getting healthy and improving your mood.* Oakland, CA: New Harbinger.

Chapter 11

Albers, S. (2012). Eating mindfully: How to end mindless eating and enjoy a balanced relationship with food (2nd ed.). Oakland, CA: New Harbinger.

Beyer, J. L., & Payne, M. E. (2016). Nutrition and bipolar depression. *Psychiatric Clinics of North America, 39*(1), 75–86.

Brown, A. J., Smith, L. T., & Craighead, L. W. (2010). Appetite awareness as a mediator in an eating disorders prevention program. *Eating Disorders, 18*(4), 286–301.

Craighead, L. W. (2006). *The appetite awareness workbook: How to listen to your body and overcome bingeing, overeating, and obsession with food.* Oakland, CA: New Harbinger.

Craighead, L. W. (2017). *Training your inner pup to eat well: Let your stomach be your guide.* Alpharetta, GA: Lanier Press.

Dsouza, A., Haque, S., & Aggarwal, R. (2019). The influence of ketogenic diets on mood stability in bipolar disorder. *Asian Journal of Psychiatry, 41*, 86–87.

Dunbar, R. I. M. (2017). Breaking bread: The functions of social eating. *Adaptive Human Behavior and Physiology, 3*(3), 198–211.

Frigerio, S., Strawbridge, R., & Young, A. H. (2021). The impact of caffeine consumption on clinical symptoms in patients with bipolar disorder: A systematic review. *Bipolar Disorders, 23*(3), 241–251.

Fung, T. T., Long, M. W., Hung, P., & Cheung, L. W. (2016). An expanded model for mindful eating for health promotion and sustainability: Issues and challenges for dietetics practice. *Journal of the Academy of Nutrition and Dietetics, 116*(7), 1081–1086.

Goehler, L. (2022). *Food for thought: Changing how we feel by changing how we eat.* New York: Institute for Disease and Disaster Management.

Kilbourne, A. M., Rofey, D. L., McCarthy, J. F., Post, E. P., Welsh, D., & Blow, F. C. (2007). Nutrition and exercise behavior among patients with bipolar disorder. *Bipolar Disorders, 9*(5), 443–452.

Luo, J., Xia, M., & Zhang, C. (2022). The effects of chewing gum on reducing anxiety and stress: A meta-analysis of randomized controlled trials. *Journal of Healthcare Engineering,* 8606693.

McElroy, S. L., Kemp, D. E., Friedman, E. S., Reilly-Harrington, N. A., Sylvia, L. G., Calabrese, J. R., . . . Shelton, R. C. (2016). Obesity, but not metabolic syndrome, negatively affects outcome in bipolar disorder. *Acta Psychiatrica Scandinavica, 133*(2), 144–153.

Miquel, S., Haddou, M. B., & Day, J. E. L. (2019). A systematic review and meta-analysis of the effects of mastication on sustained attention in healthy adults. *Physiology and Behavior, 202*, 101–115.

Thich Nhat Hanh & Cheung, L. (2010). *Savor: Mindful eating, mindful life.* San Francisco: HarperOne.

Chapter 12

Broyd, S. J., van Hell, H. H., Beale, C., Yucel, M., & Solowij, N. (2016). Acute and chronic effects of cannabinoids on human cognition—a systematic review. *Biological Psychiatry, 79*(7), 557–567.

Cerullo, M. A., & Strakowski, S. M. (2007). The prevalence and significance of substance use disorders in bipolar type I and II disorder. *Substance Abuse Treatment, Prevention, and Policy, 2,* 29.

DelBello, M. P., Strakowski, S. M., Sax, K. W., McElroy, S. L., Keck, P. E., Jr., West, S. A., & Kmetz, G. F. (1999). Familial rates of affective and substance use disorders in patients with first-episode mania. *Journal of Affective Disorders, 56*(1), 55–60.

Fusar-Poli, P., Crippa, J. A., Bhattacharyya, S., Borgwardt, S. J., Allen, P., Martin-Santos, R., . . . McGuire, P. K. (2009). Distinct effects of delta9-tetrahydrocannabinol and cannabidiol on neural activation during emotional processing. *Archives of General Psychiatry, 66*(1), 95–105.

Hjorthoj, C., Ostergaard, M. L., Benros, M. E., Toftdahl, N. G., Erlangsen, A., Andersen, J. T., & Nordentoft, M. (2015). Association between alcohol and substance use disorders and all-cause and cause-specific mortality in schizophrenia, bipolar disorder, and unipolar depression: A nationwide, prospective, register-based study. *Lancet Psychiatry, 2*(9), 801–808.

McPheeters, M., O'Connor, E. A., Riley, S., Kennedy, S. M., Voisin, C., Kuznacic, K., . . . Jonas, D. E. (2023). Pharmacotherapy for alcohol use disorder: A systematic review and meta-analysis. *JAMA, 330*(17), 1653–1665.

Pintori, N., Caria, F., De Luca, M. A., & Miliano, C. (2023). THC and CBD: Villain versus hero? Insights into adolescent exposure. *International Journal of Molecular Sciences, 24*(6), 5251.

Single, E. (1996). Harm reduction as an alcohol-prevention strategy. *Alcohol Health and Research World, 20*(4), 239–243. *www.ncbi.nlm.nih.gov/pmc/articles/PMC6876518*

Strakowski, S. M., DelBello, M. P., Fleck, D. E., Adler, C. M., Anthenelli, R. M., Keck, P. E., Jr., . . . Amicone, J. (2005). Effects of co-occurring alcohol abuse on the course of bipolar disorder following a first hospitalization for mania. *Archives of General Psychiatry, 62*(8), 851–858.

Strakowski, S. M., DelBello, M. P., Fleck, D. E., & Arndt, S. (2000). The impact of substance abuse on the course of bipolar disorder. *Biological Psychiatry, 48*(6), 477–485.

Tourjman, S. V., Buck, G., Jutras-Aswad, D., Khullar, A., McInerney, S., Saraf, G., . . . Beaulieu, S. (2023). Canadian Network for Mood and Anxiety Treatments (CANMAT) task force report: A systematic review and recommendations of cannabis use in bipolar disorder and major depressive disorder. *Candian Journal of Psychiatry, 68*(5), 299–311.

Chapter 13

American Psychiatric Association. (2022). *Diagnostic and statistical manual of mental disorders* (5th ed., text rev.). Arlington, VA: Author.

Baldessarini, R. J., Tondo, L., Ghiani, C., & Lepri, B. (2010). Illness risk following rapid versus gradual discontinuation of antidepressants. *American Journal of Psychiatry, 167*(8), 934–941.

Baldessarini, R. J., Tondo, L., & Hennen, J. (1999). Effects of lithium treatment and its discontinuation on suicidal behavior in bipolar manic-depressive disorders. *Journal of Clinical Psychiatry, 60*(Suppl. 2), 77–84.

Goldberg, J. F., DelBello, M. P., & Swartz, H. A. (2022). Expanded treatment options and addressing unmet needs in the diagnosis and treatment of bipolar disorder. *Journal of Clinical Psychiatry, 83*(6), MS21058AH5.

Hirschfeld, R. M., Lewis, L., & Vornik, L. A. (2003). Perceptions and impact of bipolar disorder: How far have we really come? Results of the National Depressive and Manic-Depressive Association 2000 Survey of Individuals with Bipolar Disorder. *Journal of Clinical Psychiatry, 64*, 161–174.

Miklowitz, D. J., & Gitlin, M. J. (2015). *Clinician's guide to bipolar disorder.* New York: Guilford Press.

Suppes, T., Baldessarini, R. J., Faedda, G. L., Tondo, L., & Tohen, M. (1993). Discontinuation of maintenance treatment in bipolar disorder: Risks and implications. *Harvard Review of Psychiatry, 1*(3), 131–144.

Chapter 14

Jamison, K. R. (1995). *An unquiet mind: A memoir of moods and madness.* New York: Knopf.

Miklowitz, D. J. (2010). *Bipolar disorder: A family-focused treatment approach* (2nd ed.). New York: Guilford Press.

Miklowitz, D. J., Efthimiou, O., Furukawa, T. A., Scott, J., McLaren, R., Geddes, J. R., & Cipriani, A. (2021). Adjunctive psychotherapies for bipolar disorder: A systematic review and component network meta-analysis. *JAMA Psychiatry, 78*(2), 141–150.

index

about the author

David J. Miklowitz, PhD, is Distinguished Professor of Psychiatry and Biobehavioral Sciences at the Semel Institute for Neuroscience and Human Behavior, David Geffen School of Medicine, University of California, Los Angeles, and Visiting Professor in the Department of Psychiatry at the University of Oxford, United Kingdom. He is the author of *The Bipolar Disorder Survival Guide,* for general readers, and several award-winning books for professionals, including *Bipolar Disorder: A Family-Focused Treatment Approach, Second Edition.* Dr. Miklowitz has published over 300 scientific articles and 70 book chapters. He has won Distinguished Investigator awards from the Brain and Behavior Research Foundation, the Depression and Bipolar Support Alliance, the International Society for Bipolar Disorders, and the Society for a Science of Clinical Psychology. Dr. Miklowitz has been appointed to endowed lectureships from the University of Oxford, Massachusetts General Hospital, the University of Massachusetts School of Medicine, and Case Western Reserve University School of Medicine. He is one of the few psychologists to have received the Award for Research in Mood Disorders from the American College of Psychiatrists.